MIDLIFE MAN

ART HISTER, MD

MIDLIFE MAN

• • •

A NOT-SO-THREATENING GUIDE TO HEALTH AND SEX FOR MAN AT HIS PEAK

GREYSTONE BOOKS
Douglas & McIntyre Publishing Group
Vancouver / Toronto / Berkeley

For Phyllis, Jonah, and Tim

First edition 1998

07 08 09 10 5 4 3 2

Greystone Books
A division of Douglas & McIntyre Ltd.
2323 Quebec Street, Suite 201
Vancouver, British Columbia
Canada V5T 4S7
www.greystonebooks.com

Library and Archives Canada Cataloguing in Publication
Hister, Art
Midlife man : a not-so-threatening guide to health and sex for man at his peak / Art Hister.—2nd ed.

Includes index.

ISBN-13: 978-1-55365-132-1 · ISBN-10: 1-55365-132-4

1. Middle-aged men—Health and hygiene. 2. Climacteric, Male. I. Title.
RA777.8.H58 2006 613′.04234 C2005-907484-1

Editing by Nancy Flight
Copy editing by Barbara Tomlin
Cover design by Naomi MacDougall
Text design by Jessica Sullivan
Front jacket photograph by Chick Rice
Printed and bound in Canada by Friesens
Printed on acid-free paper that is forest friendly (100% post-consumer recycled paper) and has been processed chlorine free.
Distributed in the U.S. by Publishers Group West

We gratefully acknowledge the financial support of the Canada Council for the Arts, the British Columbia Arts Council, and the Government of Canada through the Book Publishing Industry Development Program (BPIDP) for our publishing activities.

CONTENTS

• • •

PREFACE TO THE REVISED EDITION

• • •

The second worst thing about producing a book is that over the years some of the words and thoughts you once put into the public domain eventually come back to haunt you. The worst thing about writing a book is that what you wrote about friends and family haunts you the moment the book comes out. If you want some true enemies for life, just publish a few anecdotes—true or made-up—about your friends or, worse, your family: no extra turkey for you at family gatherings (in fact, you may not even get invited).

So, a little over seven years ago, I sat down and started writing what eventually became *Midlife Man*: the thoughts, theories, tales, and tribulations of a man who had just entered his fifties (OK, OK—so I'd actually been in my fifties for nearly three years, but like baby boomers always claim, I felt much younger than my chronological age). At the time I honestly felt on top of the world, or as close to the top as I thought I would ever get. And, I claimed, I was certainly not alone in feeling like that. Most fifty-year-old men, I wrote, "are happy and satisfied—at least as happy as they are ever going to be."

I also wrote at the time that, all variables and caveats (such as physical health, emotional well-being, financial state, and social relationships) considered, I was hoping and rather expecting that my own carefully nurtured contentment would likely continue for a few more years—something that was cause for much ridicule, by the way, among the people who know me. My wife, for one, sniffed loudly to one of our friends that "Only an idiot would be so cheery about the prospect of growing older," and that was one of her kinder contributions to that conversation.

At this point, readers of the first edition may well be wondering, "How the hell has that idiot done, anyway?" The happy answer is, "Pretty much as this idiot thought he'd do," so ha, ha, on you, you skeptics. In fact, without tempting the dybbuks that continually loiter waiting to spring unwelcome surprises on foolish, contented braggadocios, I would say that I'm doing even better than I thought I'd do, and certainly better than most of my critics had predicted I would do.

Yes, as obnoxious as this may sound, I feel just as happy with the overall state of my life as I near that watershed of sixty as I felt seven years ago, and from most more objective measures, I'm doing at least as well as I was doing back then. In fact, by many of those measures, I'm doing even better than I used to do, in large part because of the many changes in my life, some anticipated, some not, some deliberate, some not, that have transpired over the last seven years, and which I will discuss in this new edition. That's the good news.

On the downside, though, I have become prey to some physical and emotional changes that I did not expect to hit me in quite the way they did, and I have become concerned with worries that I did not expect to confront, all of which has come as rather a surprise to this know-it-all—to borrow a phrase my kids use to describe their dad.

So in this new edition for the new millennium, I will, of course, go over all the old ground I covered in the first edition, which was focussed mainly on matters affecting midlife men around the age of fifty, as well as add in heaps of new findings about health issues that have come along in the interim, such as those about erectile dysfunction and premature ejaculation and cardiac health and many other topics. But in this new edition and with this more advanced perspective, I will also discuss many of the somewhat surprising changes and worries that confront an even older midlife man.

But hey, in case some of my peers nearing sixty are worrying about where older midlife is going to take them, rest assured, guys, that I still feel a lot like that dude on the cover (from the neck down, anyway.)

INTRODUCTION

• • •

Middle age is when you're sitting at home on a Saturday night
and the telephone rings and you hope it's not for you.

OGDEN NASH

There are probably as many myths about
midlife now as there were about aging thirty years ago.

GILBERT BRIM, quoted in "Midlife Myths"
by Winifred Gallagher, *Atlantic Monthly*

I'm still not sure how the single-celled idea to write a book that was originally supposed to be titled something like *The Crumbling, Aging Male—A First-Person Perspective* came to life. But when I told my wife of this vague proposal from my publisher, she immediately said, "I can't think of anyone who would be more right to do such a book than you, dear."

Sadly, my wife was far from a lone voice. Nearly all my colleagues, most listeners to my radio show, my car mechanic, my lawyer, strangers I met in bars, indeed just about everyone who knows me at all, and some who knew me only for minutes, seemed to instantly agree that yes, I would indeed be the perfect person to write a book about "how all you guys deteriorate as you get older," as an ex-friend put it, not even bothering to suppress her smirk.

This idea, then, seemed to have "legs" right from the moment it first saw light. The clincher, however, was the regular and terribly insensitive reminders from my teenage sons that even though I had once worked at a free clinic and even though I had truly, honestly swear-to-God been at Woodstock (the original one, not the twenty-fifth anniversary ersatz one with all those balding, wrinkled, potbellied has-beens—both performers and attendees), I have indeed become, as my boys like to say, "like really old, man." So even though my thirty-year-old bell-bottoms did eventually come back into style (though clearly not on me), everyone's snide remarks finally led me to acknowledge that my days as a boy-wonder (a legend in my own mind) had indeed come and gone. I have been forced to recognize that I am well into the next phase of my life, a recognition shoved in my face a few years ago when, along with twenty thousand others of my generation, I attended a Van Morrison–Joni Mitchell–Bob Dylan last-hurrah concert. Now that I have become a committed middle-aged nonsmoker, when it came time for the audience to wave its lighters during a particularly nostalgic number, I waved my cellular phone instead. And so did most of the people around me.

"So why not write about it," I asked myself. "Especially since the publisher has been dumb enough to give me an advance, meagre though it is." Besides, I reasoned further, maybe I have a duty to write this book, to let my fellow aging brothers, and especially their spouses and inheritors, know that at the age of fifty, a male is not necessarily so close to death that he can feel the Grim Reaper's hot breath on his neck.

Having seen this milestone come and go, I have become convinced that a man at fifty is still quite young. And because of medical advances, as well as the fact that those of us now entering our sixth decade have by and large lived a much healthier life than our fathers did, many more of us near-geezers will live into our eighties and nineties than ever before, a thought that no doubt terrifies our inheritors. And they may have a bit of a point because God only knows how society will handle a world overrun with shrivelled, slippered, unshaven, leaky ninety-year-old men. For a start, they're going to have to build a lot more sit-down spaces and bathrooms in the malls. At that Morrison–Mitchell–Dylan concert, for example, the lineups in the men's washrooms were out the door, as all the old farts seemed to take forever to get their business done.

This book, then, is about middle age in a male: his fantasies, his fears, his failures, his frustrations, his physical falloff, his finagling, and his future, and my purpose is to let every man over forty know what to expect as he plunges into the coming two decades. But because I have learned over the years that the average guy would rather bring Martha Stewart or Roseanne home to meet his mom and dad than admit that he wants or needs to find out more about his health, I also intend this book to be read by women who live with, work with, or deal with men. Not only do I hope this book will help such women understand what is happening to old lifeless lard-butt, who prefers to sit in his living room soaking up the suds rather than to sit on his cycle sweating off the suet, but I also hope that many women will read appropriate sections of this text aloud to their mates or male colleagues and thus perhaps prompt them to read it on their own, and maybe even goad them into doing something with the information.

"But," many of you are probably wondering, "aside from your need to write it and your wish to make a few extra bucks, Art, why is a book like this really necessary? After all, we have all those health shows on television and radio to tell us about this stuff."

Over the last few years we have indeed witnessed a rapidly growing interest in health and a corresponding explosion of investigative programs as well as open-mouth television and radio shows (one of which I host, by the way—consult your local listings for the time in your area, and if you can't find a listing, bug your local station to pick up this excellent show) to cater to this interest. The problem, however, is that such programs, governed as they all are by the ratings they draw and little else, are by their very nature both superficial and sensation seeking. So if, for example, you would like to know how and why so many left-handed cross-dressing transsexuals have murdered their lesbian lovers in midlife, television will undoubtedly be happy to provide you with the answer, and I'm sure it has already done so. But if you would like to know in some depth what happens to normal middle-aged men (not an oxymoron, by the way), there is little reliable, verifiable, and accessible information available to you, and much of what is available is often more myth or wishful thinking than reality.

This paucity of information about middle-aged men stands in stark contrast to what we know about women and middle age. As anyone with an interest in health can attest, these days women approaching menopause are the medical, social, cultural, political, even economic flavour du jour. Consequently, we are all deluged daily with data about menopause-related changes, what choices women can make to ease this passage, how long they will suffer with the symptoms, and how they are likely to fare. Every day, it seems, spawns yet another article or a new finding about menopause, which is why a typical man probably knows more about what estrogen can do for hot flashes and vaginal dryness than he does about what finasteride can do for his swollen prostate.

Now please note that I am not at all blaming menopausal women for this disparity, mostly because, for personal reasons, I would never dare do that. I value my well-being, and my place in bed. It's not women's fault that men have so little information about themselves. No, the fault for that, I'm afraid, resides nearly entirely with men themselves. The sad truth is that in the past, most men, but especially younger ones, were clearly not much interested in their bodies, particularly in its failings.

To be fair, the reason for this lack of concern about health matters stems from the average younger man's generally happy physiological state, because if he is born healthy and he can avoid getting into accidents and developing chronic illnesses, very little generally goes wrong to disturb the average under-forty-year-old man's normal condition of intact wellness and his corresponding state of blissful and willful medical ignorance.

So while from a rather early age on women are constantly reminded of their oh-so-changeable bodies—surviving periods, pregnancies, parturition, and more—a typically clueless and average man can swing along from the time he starts to shave until the time he is getting up twice a night to pee and never notice a change in how his body functions. In addition, when a medical problem does crop up, the typical male reacts in one of two ways. He tends either to deny that there is anything wrong until it can no longer be avoided ("You know, George, you really should have come to see me before this lump got to be the size of a grapefruit." "I know, doc, only I was sure it would go away on its own.") or else he panics and immediately presumes the worst. To most men, nearly every cough represents a budding pneumonia and every two-day headache heralds a brain tumour, until proven otherwise. Happily, such proof can generally be offered in short order by a wife who says, "Grow up. It's only a cold." The physiological constancy of their bodies married to men's natural aversion to knowing more about their health bred an understandable medical nonchalance and lack of curiosity in the men who came before my generation.

Science obliged men who did not want to know more by not doing much research on the normal events that happen to healthy men. Thus, we know a great deal about old men; we know a great deal about boys; we know the most about sick men. But we really don't know much about what normal, middle-aged men should expect or do.

Things are changing, however. Prompted by the example of baby-boomer women, who have prodded and persuaded the medical world to find answers for what is happening to their bodies at every stage of their lives—from the time they are fetuses in utero, when they first begin to move their jaws way more than their male counterparts do (it's true, and I am smart enough and scared enough to make no editorial comment about that) to the time they finally rejoin their husbands, who predeceased them, in happy eternal interment—many male members of the most narcissistic, self-involved generation to have ever come along (until Generation X got here, of course; now there is a bunch of crybabies sans peer) have also taken an increasing interest in their bodies. These men have begun to bleat loudly, as only baby boomers can do, that they want answers about what is happening to them right now, what is likely to happen to them in the near future, and what they can do about stopping it.

To silence those lambs, I am happy to say that we are now seeing an increasing amount of attention paid to the health concerns of normal midlife men, especially to what some researchers call andropause or viropause, the so-called male menopause. We have also witnessed a corresponding outpouring of headline-grabbing findings about this newly discovered and seemingly inevitable passage in every man's life.

As always, though, the headlines don't tell the whole story. Is there really reliable evidence that a universal and inevitable metabolic or hormonal change affects all men at a certain time in life? And what about the infamous "male midlife crisis," a rather indistinct term referring to a cataclysmic event that presumably stems from ennui or fear. Is a midlife crisis really inevitable, or is it simply the product of some overeager Hollywood scriptwriters' imaginations? Is every wife doomed to wake up one day to find her trusty five-year-old, seven-seater Dodge van replaced by a two-seater silver Porsche in her driveway? (And who is most likely to occupy that second seat?) Or worse, is every Brittany and Chelsea and Tiffany a potential stepmom to every menopausal Mary's or Jan's or Linda's kids? Should every aging libidinally challenged man start taking testosterone as hormone replacement therapy? Should his spouse do the same? And what about Viagra? Is it really the answer to all your drooping dreams? Are Viagrified men the new Godzillas—hairy, fearsome, and on the prowl? You'll have to read on to find out, I'm afraid.

But one last word before you do. If you are looking for cheap jokes and sad endings, you will be disappointed. The cheap jokes are here in abundance, of course. I'm a Jewish Canadian male, after all. That's the only way we know how to survive.

The sad ending, however, is not here. You see, I strongly disagree with those authors, the newly minted minions of male menopause mavens, who claim that despite their outward bravado, nearly all middle-aged men are silently unhappy creatures, terrified of losing their youth and petrified of old age. I do not agree, as so many authors seem to claim, that most middle-aged men are desperate to find a way out of their caught-in-the-middle position (no longer man-on-the-way-up, not yet man-on-the-way-out), frantically seeking equally unhappy brothers with whom they can go into the woods, wrestle in the mud, cry together over a few beers or herbal tea, and beat some drums.

Rather, I believe that middle age is a great time of life, a time when most of us, men and women both, finally feel as if we're on top of whatever hill we had set out to climb so many years ago (or at least as close to the top as we're ever likely to get, given how out of breath many of us become these days when we do any climbing). I also believe that middle age is that time of life when we are most flexible and most able to roll with the punches life inevitably hits us with. Middle age is when we are most able to accommodate those changes that will allow us to be what we want to be when we finally grow up.

I believe that for many men, probably most men, what happens to us in midlife is not nearly as unwelcome as we have been led to believe. For most of us, midlife is the best time of life, and many of the changes that accompany middle age are not only pleasant but the harbingers of even better things to come.

So be warned by a man who drives a dented, seven-year-old SUV (I'm probably too fat to fit comfortably into a small sports car, my bad back won't let me bend that far, and besides, for a Jewish man, there are way too many gears in those vroom boxes). Middle age is not the beginning of the end. Most men come through their middle years happy with themselves and with their lives, proud of their achievements, valued by their families and society in general, and determined to make the second half of their lives even better and richer. Although I must ruefully acknowledge, as most of my peers must too, that many of the goals I had set myself in my younger years will never be achieved (I will never figure out how a carburetor works or even what it is, I will never ski a double-black-diamond run—in fact, I may never even get down a blue run in one schuss—and I will certainly never play the piano for the symphony, in part because I will probably never even learn to play the piano unless I take a few lessons), I also believe that in many other very important respects, for me and for most midlife men, the present is pleasant, perhaps even the best there is, and the next few years promise to be just as good.

{1}

THAT WAS THEN—THIS IS NOW

• • •

If youth's theme is potential, midlife's is reality: childhood fantasies are past, the fond remembrances of age are yet to be, and the focus is on coming to terms with the finite resources of the here and now. The overwhelming majority... accomplish this developmental task... through a long, gentle process...

WINIFRED GALLAGHER, "Midlife Myths," *Atlantic Monthly*

Midlife is the black box of human development...

DR. ORVILLE GILBERT BRIM, Director of the MacArthur Foundation Research Network on Successful Midlife Development

There was a time, I remember, when my hair did not plug up the drain after every shower, when my knees did not make those high-pitched, loose-board creaks they now emit each morning as I take my first steps, when I needed only one pair of unifocal glasses, when the pain from even a severely pulled muscle lasted no more than a few days and required no more therapy than my old standby typical-male remedy of feeling extremely sorry for myself. Back then, I never hesitated to bend down to pick up an object on the ground or help a friend move his household goods or try to open the lid of a virgin pickle jar using only my still-firm hands.

I also remember when I could still eat huge quantities of food and lie down immediately afterwards without worrying about how this activity would affect my belt line or how far up the esophagus my overly adventurous digestive juices would burn. Back in those days, I could still devour mounds and mounds of several kinds of garlic sausage, the amount limited only by my consideration for the company I would have to face following the meal, and I could still drink as much alcohol as I could afford to buy or, better yet, have bought for me.

That was oh so long ago now, when I didn't yet need gingko biloba or other supplements to stimulate my memory (at least I think it's gingko biloba I'm taking for my memory, because honestly, I can't remember which of the several "G" supplements—gingko, garlic, glucosamine, ginger, ginseng—I should be taking and for which conditions).

I am even more changed now than when I wrote *Midlife Man* in the 1990s. I am now, alas, fairly close to that character of ridicule—the aging, balding, grinning white guy, who desperately tries every combing technique known to man to evenly distribute his remaining three thin hairs across the moonscape of his skull. And those many new tufts of non-skull hair that had started sprouting a few years ago have, as expected, continued to proliferate and worse, to burst forth gloriously from ever-more numerous and previously hair-free portals to my body. On the positive side, my ocular needs have stabilized and my trifocals are still sufficient to help me see most objects, although I still can't read very well unless the page is held at exactly the right distance from my eyes.

Still on the positive side, my previously chronically hurting back hurts far less often than it once did, in large part because about six years ago I started a vigorous exercise regimen (you can—and should—read all about it in my other best seller, *Dr. Art Hister's Guide to Living a Long and Healthy Life*), so that I am now the owner of a few palpable muscles, the first stirrings of what are known in the fitness world as "abs," and other "core" muscles that have taken lots of strain off my back and greatly reduced the number of times I end up with back pain.

And still with positive news about my changes since the first edition of *Midlife Man* (I know you are holding your breath in anticipation), my exercise program has markedly shrunk my bulging midriff. Yes, I still own an equatorial protrusion that keeps me from endlessly admiring my profile in front of the mirror (after all, exercise can't produce miracles), but it has shrunk noticeably (think hillock rather than domed stadium), and overall I've lost about thirty-five pounds since I wrote *Midlife Man*—not bad for a man at this stage of life, eh?

On the negative side, however, despite my new health regimen, the gastroesophageal reflux disease that I have suffered from for years has continued to be a real bother so that I've moved beyond a bottle of extra-strength, double-duty antacid tablets (which can, however, still be found at my bedside for regular nightly use), and I now have to take an even more potent form of antiacid medication to control my refluxing acid problem (acids, like kids and dogs, love going places they were never invited to visit).

Also, as you'd expect from an aging male, I've had absolutely no relief from my overactive bladder and ever-expanding prostate, so that more than ever I have to think very carefully about how much and what kind of liquids I consume before going to a movie or getting on a plane in case I don't get an aisle seat. For a midlife man, hell is a window seat in economy class next to Martha Stewart on a plane delayed on takeoff (although I very much doubt that Martha would ever be caught dead in economy class, not unless she could redesign the seats and plastic cutlery).

Moreover, gravity's continuing unfettered run at imposing its control on my naïve tissues has led most of my external parts, as well as a few internal ones, to slither even lower (in some cases, it's well beyond slithering; "plunging" would be more appropriate). Worse, some of me has also continued to shrink even more, and since I'm only five foot six (perhaps even five foot five now, although I refuse to verify that), I don't really have much to give back. Worst of all, though, some of me has begun to deteriorate, and as an added indignity, some of my parts have even started to hurt occasionally without any evident provocation. When provoked, they hurt even more and for longer.

So what has happened to me? Without realizing it, without expecting it, and certainly without welcoming it, I have become even more my father: balding, bulging, buckling, belching, braying, and beyond forty. It's gone so far that I have even (Oh, the shame of admitting it!) bought a recliner. Even worse, I've actually gone on a genuine honest to goodness packed with over eaters cruise. True, I didn't much like the cruise, but hey, that doesn't really matter, does it? After all, I was there on deck—more accurately, in the dining room—with those other middle-aged potbellies, sidling up to the midnight snack bar and mumbling about how bad this must be for my health, but oh, the cheesecake! And—horrors for my wife!—I have now on several occasions worn long underwear on what threatened to be cool days—in July. (But then, so has she.)

But here's the thing: in my generation I am certainly not an exception. All of us middle-agers are suffering these bodily insults and alarming symptoms of premature old fogeyness, and most guys I know have become quite altered—physically, emotionally, spiritually, even financially—in the last few years.

This is nothing new, of course. Similar profound changes happened to our fathers, and to their fathers, and to all the fathers that came before them.

What is new, however, is that unlike our dads who took everything in stride without asking questions ("Sure, doc, I'll take eight of those mango-sized pills every day, and no, I don't really care to know why you gave them to me. You're the doctor, after all."), an increasing number of us middle-aged gents want to know what these changes portend and how our likely ends can be, if not permanently postponed, at least substantially delayed. Which changes are normal? Which changes are warning signals of impending physical or emotional disaster? Most important, what can we do about them? How can we prevent them? Can we even delay, dare I mention His Name (I'll whisper it), Death? Where can we run to? And where can we hide?

The difficulty with answering these questions, however, is that as I first wrote seven years ago, midlife for men is still a largely unstudied period, and we males are about twenty years behind our female counterparts in what science can tell us about what is normal in middle age. Although this state of affairs is changing, and men's midlife hormonal, psychological, and emotional changes are now the subject of many studies, most of these studies have not been completed, so we are still left with much speculation.

Hot Flash! A Male Menopause?

About the only comfort all the other guys my age and I can draw from the many changes we are enduring is the knowledge that they are not confined to men. Middle-aged women also undergo profound physical changes, but happily for them, women can at least attribute many of their symptoms to a defined, measurable, universally recognized, hormonal change: menopause. And although hormone replacement therapy (HRT) has fallen into much well-earned disrepute, women who have a very bumpy ride through menopause can at least allay some of the worst symptoms with HRT. What is not generally known, however, is that many midlife men experience many of the same outrageous slings and symptoms that affect women going through menopause. No, men don't get vaginal dryness, but many of us do suffer from mood swings, increased anxiety, back pain, insomnia, headaches, and even hot flashes. The difference between the genders, however, is this: science has still not established that in midlife men these symptoms are produced by hormonal changes, nor that a drop in hormone levels with age, which all men do experience, has much effect on men, nor that most men require or are helped by hormonal intervention for those common symptoms.

On one level, then, that makes the issue of whether men suffer a menopause rather cut-and-dried. If we adopt a narrow definition of menopause as simply "the cessation of menstruation, and by extension, the cessation of natural reproductive ability," men clearly do not go through a male equivalent of menopause. So although a man's reproductive capacity diminishes with age, as so many men from our biblical forefathers Jacob and Abraham to Pablo Picasso and Rod Stewart have exuberantly and visibly demonstrated, a man's ability to impregnate a partner—naturally—can stay intact until an older age, and as abhorrent as the thought may be to most of us, some very old men can and do sire inheritors. At least that's the story their much younger wives inevitably tell them. I mean, without DNA testing, who knows who Isaac's father really was? Hey, maybe we're all half-Jewish.

But such a narrow definition of menopause drastically misses the mark, I think, because for women, menopause is much more than a time when hormone levels drop and periods peter out and birth control ceases to be a worry. The several years that make up the perimenopausal and menopausal period are also a time of great upheaval and change—physical, emotional, psychological, economic, and spiritual—in almost every woman's life, a time when so much more than just her reproductive abilities are altered.

Middle-aged men experience these changes too. Most noticeably, our bodies change significantly, and these alterations are visible not only to ourselves but to anyone unlucky enough to see us in the full or even half Monty. Just as important, our emotions also go through adjustments in midlife, often dramatically, our spiritual needs often shift significantly, and our social and employment status is also often affected.

If, then, we take a broader perspective consistent with the more realistic and less restrictive worldview most of us have probably developed by our less liberal middle years (after all, isn't midlife the time for admitting that concrete really is much more appealing than unmowed brown grass, and that the only Buffet we should have listened to in our younger years was Warren, not Jimmy), we can also learn to accept a much wider definition of menopause, one that applies to men as well as women.

A very good example of such a definition can be found in Jed Diamond's book *Male Menopause*. "*Male menopause*," writes Diamond, "begins with hormonal, physiological, and chemical changes that occur in all men between the ages of forty and fifty-five... These changes affect all aspects of a man's life. Male menopause is, thus, a physical condition with psychological, interpersonal, social, and spiritual dimensions."

I agree completely with Diamond. I believe the term "menopause," whether we apply it to men or to women, should not be restricted to hormonal changes only but rather should signify a universal passage during midlife that encompasses hormonal, physiological, emotional, biochemical, psychological, and spiritual changes that are linked to corresponding alterations in health, outlook, expectations, self-perception, relationships, family ties, and social status. Although much more Histerian—that is, long-winded, complex, and easily forgotten—this latter definition is a great deal more consistent with what we now know happens during midlife to all men and women.

But here's that gender difference again: taking into account our knowledge of hormones today (and there is no doubt that we will find many new hormones in the future), we can also conclude that what happens to most middle-aged men is not nearly as hormonally driven or directed as the passage that middle-aged women go through or that the common use of the term menopause implies. (In fact, that is why many experts now prefer to call this change of life in men andropause or viropause rather than male menopause.) Indeed, it can easily be argued that for most males, adolescence (and perhaps old age too) is a much more turbulent, hormonally driven period than is midlife.

So here's the bottom line: midlife for men is not a time of dramatic hormonal changes. Yes, it can be volcanic, but the vast majority of midlife men, I submit, are generally happy souls, busily navigating, to the best of our often amateurish and certainly friable abilities, an occasionally uneven continuum from early adulthood to slipperhood. And the great thing is that we usually manage to navigate safely, getting bruised a bit on the way, to be sure, but surviving largely intact, full sails up. Yes, it often takes midlife man a bit longer to get his sails up than it used to, and sometimes he can't even get them up at all or at best only to quarter-mast, but he knows that if he just waits a day or two or sometimes seven—or if he just takes certain pills, one of which is heavily promoted by an ex-candidate for president of the United States of America—the wind will surely return, and then it's full mast again, for one quick sailing at least.

Our Need to Medicalize Everything

If there is little proof that midlife men undergo a dramatic hormonal change, why, you may wonder, is there so much interest in establishing a hormonally based "male menopause"? That one is easy to answer. It's largely because of Western medicine's push to medicalize everything to do with health and well-being, because the more aspects of our lives that doctors and other health professionals can claim is a deviation from some norm, the more they can treat (some might say interfere with or control, but hey, I would never say that). And coming up with new syndromes and conditions gives much work to many people who might otherwise just be greeting shoppers at Wal-Mart. What's worse is that many of these self-appointed buttinskies don't seem to care that there is very little universal agreement or even consensus about what constitutes a normal level of so many behaviours, whims, conditions, choices, habits, vapours, actions, hormones, cell counts, and even symptoms, yet are still prepared to rush in with some type of intervention if they think someone or something is not "normal." So in this treatment-first world, mild sadness becomes "depression," shyness is re-named "social anxiety syndrome," normal aging in men is turned into "andropause," and so on. In fact, one recent report concluded that the majority of us will eventually develop some form of "mental illness." In other words, according to these experts, most of you are now nuts (I'm clearly in the minority), although when you look around, maybe that's not such a wild theory. Now, I can handle the fact that there are a lot more forms of mild illness than were ever dreamt of in our philosophies. What I can't handle is the fact that each of these incarnations begets a bevy of new and expensive treatments, no matter how flimsy the evidence is and no matter how poor the proof that the interventions even work. It's not that these interventionists mean harm: it's that they leap before looking and thus often err on the side of over-interference. Often the associations doctors make between their observations and their calculations are tenuous at best and dangerous and misleading at worst, as is evident from a favourite old joke of mine. A scientist captures a frog. He tells the frog to jump, and the frog leaps four feet. He then cuts off one of the frog's legs and again tells the frog to jump. The frog now jumps three feet. The scientist then cuts off another leg and so on until the frog has no legs. "Jump," says the august investigator. The frog doesn't move. Again the scientist says, "Jump." The frog doesn't move. The scientist then publishes his study in a much respected journal with the conclusion that frogs with no legs are deaf. Sadly, there seem to be lots of deaf frogs out there. Deaf Frog Syndrome is a result of observer bias and merely reflects the fact that scientists are very much like everyone else—far too often, they see what they want to see.

One stark and significant real-life example of Deaf Frog Syndrome is the decades-old phenomenon in which so many exuberant and highly energetic kids, especially boys, are diagnosed with attention deficit hyperactivity disorder (ADHD) and are prescribed medications for years, many even for life (since no one has yet shown that you can really outgrow ADHD), although a diagnosis of ADHD in a particular child is often based on very questionable criteria. After all, no one has scientifically determined the limits of the continuum of "normal" behaviour, so that an observer who doesn't buy into this epidemic of ADHD could easily argue that many ADHD boys in a forty-kid classroom are probably normal, precocious, energetic boys in an environment where their exuberance is seen as disruptive.

Having been a very active boy myself, one who would no doubt be highly medicated today, I believe that many boys are being treated for just being boys, which will clearly have serious consequences for these drugged children, who will grow up not being allowed to feel and behave in what is a normal fashion for them. (Curiously, but not unexpectedly, girls who daydream are now being diagnosed in increasing numbers with ADD—attention deficit disorder without the hyperactivity component. Why limit treatment to only one gender when you can treat everyone?)

In a similar vein, a couple of decades ago the Western medical community turned its huge guns on menopause, a life passage that in most other cultures is considered a normal physiological event best left to nature, the counsel of wise women who have been there and done that, and the occasional herbal remedy. And as a consequence, an army of doctors and other self-styled experts began to urge, indeed heavily push, more than half the world's population to consider this inevitable passage to be a diseased state of hormone "deficiency" requiring urgent therapeutic intervention, not only for a few years but often for the rest of their lives.

As we now know, that push to get every perimenopausal woman to take hormones was, well, dead wrong. When researchers finally did a study that actually measured the benefits and drawbacks of hormone replacement therapy (HRT), this use of estrogen and progesterone was found to (and this is not too harsh a term) kill a lot of women who likely would have lived longer if they hadn't been exposed to our "best medical therapy" of the time.

Yet even with that stark and recent deadly wrong example in front of them, ever-growing battalions of researchers and experts are trying to do the same to men. To no one's real surprise, some researchers are finding hormonal changes in aging men that are very similiar to those found in women, and which, they claim, also require urgent medical attention. Specifically, some andrologists claim to have unearthed a small but growing community of middle-aged men whose many symptoms and health problems improve dramatically when they are placed on hormone replacement therapy consisting of testosterone and, increasingly, other androgenic hormones. The leap that these experts want the rest of us to make is that as a result of those small (and biased) samples, aging men should be taking hormone replacement therapy for the last few decades of their lives.

To be sure, research reveals that most men do suffer a plethora of vague complaints as we go through middle age. You don't have to be a brilliant researcher to discover that at fifty and at sixty we men are all much more tired than we were at twenty (I'm even more tired this week than I was last week), that all of our energies—sexual, emotional, physical, social—are not what they were when we were younger bucks, that we no longer heal as quickly as we used to, that we are more disabled by colds and flus and other transitory conditions than we once were (at least we complain more than we used to), that it now takes us longer to get going in the morning and longer to get to sleep, and that our memories and ability to concentrate are on a downhill course (I actually forgot what I was trying to say in this paragraph. Twice!).

So based on the universality of these changes, some experts have concluded that these symptoms should be lumped into a distinct syndrome called PADAM, which stands for partial androgen deficiency in the aging male, or ADAM, which is androgen deficit in the aging male. And since the symptoms are so common, most aging men, according to these experts, are now suffering from PADAM and should be treated.

The problem is that sticking several common symptoms together and calling them a "syndrome" never makes it so. Even more important, just because you may have a syndrome doesn't mean you actually need to treat it. Rather, it's incumbent on scientists to prove in randomized placebo-controlled trials that the treatment they're touting does more good than harm, not just that the treatment makes some people feel better. All treatments will make some people feel better—that's called the placebo effect. When unbiased trials are done (and they haven't been for testosterone replacement therapy), it often comes as a shock that the touted benefits of the treatments don't occur to nearly the extent promised in early, biased trials, not to mention that sometimes the treatments actually do much more harm than good, as in the case of HRT for women.

And so, I submit, this is what is happening with andropause, PADAM, BAM-BAM, or whatever you want to call aging symptoms in a normal male. (My wife has her own name for it, alte kacker kvetching disease—"alte kacker" is an old fart and "kvetching" needs no translation—and you don't have to be

Jewish to suffer from it, although it certainly helps.) No one has proved to my satisfaction that PADAM exists on a wide scale, or that most men need treatment for their symptoms, or that we know what the best therapy is for those symptoms. More important, no one has proved that the treatments in current use are safe enough in the long term to justify the wide experiment that sees many men taking testosterone replacement therapy.

Bottom line: I believe that except for a small minority of men who suffer a sharp, measurable drop in hormone levels with age, there is absolutely no proof that the symptoms of aging are associated with a fall in hormone levels in most men. Much more important, I don't believe that it has been clearly established that treating such symptoms with specific hormones will lead to more benefit than harm.

Midlife Crisis—Is a Change of Wife Inevitable?

But what about those notorious men who do flip out in middle age, the guys who are said to suffer a "midlife crisis," which has long been ascribed to a sudden hormonal hurricane that often leads directly to liposuction, a hair transplant, courses in solo sailing and paragliding, a souped-up overpriced sports car, and the overthrow of a stable, long-term marriage to someone named Anne or Nancy for a fling with Kimberly or Brittany or Chelsea, a twenty-something gum-chewing Christina Aguilera clone? Isn't the Hollywood-endorsed male midlife crisis a universal, hormonally based phenomenon that all men (and their partners) must endure? Aren't all marriages, formalized in religious ceremonies or not, threatened by a panicky midlife male fleeing his newly recognized coop? Certainly this is a common view. But is it the right one?

In a word, no. Not only is there no proof of a link between hormone changes and midlife crisis, but research also indicates that although all men (and women) go through a reassessment of their lives and life's goals during their middle years, only a small minority of men go through a significant and turbulent midlife crisis. On the contrary, midlife seems to be a balanced and even tame time for most men and their relationships. One expert, Dr. Larry Bumpass, has written that "midlife is a time of relative stability in marital status as most marriages and marital disruptions precede midlife and most widowhood occurs at older ages" (I don't know about you, but I for one was very happy to read that last bit about widowhood occurring later). Research from the American-based John D. and Catherine T. MacArthur Foundation Research Network on Successful Midlife Development (MIDMAC), one of the few institutions that has studied midlife adults, indicates that only about 5 to 10 per cent of men have a true midlife crisis. In fact, a recent book has claimed that 25 per cent of both men and women suffer midlife crises, but that was based on people's assessments of their own lives, and clearly a crisis for some people is merely a humdrum experience in the eyes of more objective observers. No matter the numbers, though, the evidence is still that it's a small minority of people who experience a profound life-altering upheaval in middle age.

It is also important to note that in many cases this self-diagnosed crisis actually had little to do with the changes that can be ascribed to midlife. In other words, many of those men were heading for trouble anyway and their crises just happened to coincide with midlife. What might be even more reassuring to most wives, though, as they weigh up old Joe over there waiting patiently behind his kids for his turn in the communal can, is that the men who do suffer a midlife crisis are usually not average Joes either. Researchers describe them as guys who tend to be selfish and immature, the kind of guys who weigh everything according to how it affects them ("But enough about me. Let's talk about you now. So tell me, what do you think about me?"), and who often hate dealing with personal or family problems. Instead of confronting an uncomfortable interpersonal situation, especially at home, these guys prefer to run away from it. (Although, to be honest can you even imagine a male who doesn't want to deal right away with a problem his wife confronts him with? Unheard of!) Thus, reports Winifred Gallagher in *Atlantic Monthly*, "people [read: men] prone to mid-life crisis score low on tests of introspection, or reflecting on one's self and on life, and high in denial, or coping with trouble by not thinking about it." In other words, these are often guys who are predestined for trouble, if not in midlife, then later on for sure. And it has very little to do with hormone swings.

It also, of course, helps if they can afford to not think about it. It's not a fluke, I think, that so many of the men who suffer severe upheavals in midlife are men with enough money to buy themselves fancy gadgets and giggling Gidgets to try to stem the perceived ebb of their manhood. Even for those guys, though—that minority of men who do endure an obvious midlife crisis—there is no credible evidence to link this "tohu vabohu" with a hormonal brownout related to their age.

So what does happen to a man in middle age? And how do most of us handle it? Well, according to Edward Young, "At thirty, man suspects himself a fool; /Knows it at forty, and reforms his plan."

Man Looking Up

Perhaps the best way to start this discussion is with a description of the typical man's life as he stands on the verge of middle age. Thus, a man in his early or mid-thirties no longer believes he will live forever, but he also has not yet acknowledged that this is really all there is. A guy in his thirties is still under the illusion that he will undoubtedly realize all those conquering dreams he has, that his magnificent talents will indeed be acknowledged one day and that he will assuredly rise considerably higher in the employment pecking order, that he will sans doubt be able to retire before he's an old geezer of sixty, that even in his sixties, he will still be making love to his spouse (her or him) several times a night—every night—on the kitchen counter (which, by the way, is why I never accept dinner invitations from young friends, although my wife says that's more because they never invite me; she may be right but I wouldn't go anyway), that his kids (many still sperm 'n' eggs) will unquestionably grow up to play for both the Yankees and the symphony, and that if he has the time and the will, he might one day allow his name to be entered as a candidate for head of state, or even better, head of the NBA or NFL (but never the NHL—not worth the headaches).

In short, a man in his thirties hasn't grown up yet, and his health and various energies have not started to decline.

That's the best part of being a thirty-something: our grandest dreams are still largely intact, even though our instincts, our spouses, and our mothers have begun to whisper otherwise, and we generally still have the energy and well-being to go after everything we want to pursue. The bad news is that a man within hailing distance of forty is also often submerged under a great deal of stress on all fronts—from his job, from his creditors, from his still meagre income and savings, from his kids, from his parents and in-laws, and most, perhaps, from his own expectations.

Then comes the reality-check of forty. Forty hits men like a ton of bricks because it is the age when most men first notice that they really do look an awful lot like their fathers ("Wow! How did that ever happen, dude?"); when they first reluctantly begin to accept that the growing layer of fat around their middles will never really melt and that they are doomed from now on to resemble buoys more than boys; when they realize that "the legs" just don't have it anymore and that it's surely time to start playing in the non-checking oldtimers' league; when they become aware—from the multiple giggles and smirks—that, on the dance floor, they now look like those cheesy old men with sucked in lower lips they had always derided for working so hard at trying to look like younger studs; when they have to acknowledge that those bald spots on their heads are not going to shrink but will instead soon resemble helicopter landing pads; when they first realize that Time's winged chariot is closing far too fast (and if you are wondering why a weekly news magazine would send out chariots to pursue anyone, you really should have paid more attention in your high school English class).

Forty, then, is when most men stop looking in mirrors and when they stop taking hits. In short, forty is when men finally start to grow up.

Unfortunately, it takes many men several years to get used to the idea that they are no longer young bucks with unlimited potential. This doesn't mean that during that time they are constantly lamenting their lost youth or anxiously contemplating their mortality. It does mean, though, for many men entering their forties, that their emotional and psychological well-being becomes shakier. After all, at forty, most of us are still physically healthy and probably at or near our peak earning capacity, so we should be feeling great about ourselves. But for many men, the cosmetic wallop that forty kicks us with, the chop to the head and the hit in the hamstrings, can significantly dampen the seemingly good fortune of being a forty-year-old in charge.

Man at His Peak

Once we accept that turn in our lives, however, most of us seem to come out of it feeling pretty good about ourselves. In fact, fifty-year-old men are the self-assessed happiest demographic group. ("Only because every idiot thinks he's happy," says my wife, but I choose to ignore that assessment. What does she know about research anyway?) According to data from Statistics Canada, for example, men (and women) between forty-five and sixty-four were most likely of all the demographic groups to claim a "high level of psychological well-being." And a National Center for Health Statistics survey of 44,000 Americans found that the happiest Americans were white middle-aged males living in the suburbs. This satisfaction with themselves (Smugness? Us?) also makes midlifers into nicer people. Thus, scientists have found that something they call "agreeableness" is highest in people in their forties, in part because they become much less extroverted as they age. Quite agree, quite agree.

But what, you may wonder, is this "high level of psychological well-being" that midlifers score highest in? According to the MIDMAC folks cited earlier:

> There are six components of psychological well-being. These are having a positive attitude toward oneself and one's past life (self-acceptance), having goals and objectives that give life meaning (purpose in life), being able to manage complex demands of daily life (environmental mastery), having a sense of continued development and self-realization (personal growth), possessing caring and trusting ties with others... and being able to follow one's own convictions.

But that still raises this key question: why are these elements of psychological health most in balance at midlife? No, it's not, as my son has theorized, that so many midlife men are on mood-altering drugs. Rather, it's because midlifers are in control, and happy to be so.

Midlife man usually has as much control over the social and economic aspects of his life and over his relationships as he is ever likely to have, and control, most experts now believe, is the real key to happiness, even, interestingly, if your health is poor. Thus, a study from Sweden concludes that even for those in their eighties and nineties, "physical frailty can be offset by an undimmed sense of mastery" or "the feeling of being actively in charge of your own life." And if this is true for ninety-year-old Swedes, it's also certainly true for fifty-year-old Canadians.

The control that midlife man exerts over his life is manifested in many ways. For example, contrary to the common view that many marriages stay intact only until the kids leave home and then the male partner also departs to link up with his true soulmate—someone half his age whom he met recently and who has never heard of Beowulf or George Orwell but who knows everything there is to know about Beyonce and Nickelback—if you're still married when you're fifty, research shows that your marriage has either begun to improve or else it's likely to do so soon. Why? Because by age fifty or so, midlife man's partner has often gone through a transition similar to his and is just as eager to get on with the rest of his or her life.

In addition, if midlife man has had kids, they are probably now at that stage where he is either about to pack them off or he already has packed them off (many have, of course, stormed off or sneaked off on their own), thus reinvigorating his relationship with his partner, and if the kids' departure doesn't always reinvigorate the relationship, then it at least allows the couple more time and energy to work things out. Men, after all, are notorious for slipping away, for avoiding confrontation, for retreating when any opportunity presents itself to march in a backwards direction, something that's always possible when kids are around, and most men would prefer to let marital conflicts fester, in the hope that they (the conflicts, not the men) will wither and die. It is, however, much harder to avoid confronting a marital problem when there are only the two of you in the house. Thus, studies show that in midlife most marital disputes tend to be settled earlier and more quickly than they used to be and without becoming as corrosive as early marriage disagreements can get. In fact, a recent study has concluded that older partners are significantly less interested in "winning" an argument than younger partners are (clearly, these researchers never met my wife), while another concluded that the older we get, the more we tend to see "the big picture," meaning that as you age, you're not as concerned any longer with winning each individual point or argument so you don't invest as much anger and hostility in disputes with your partner (although being more concerned with the "big picture" may also mean that you simply become more interested in just outlasting the other party). This state of affairs not only enhances the marriage but is also ultimately much better for a man's health.

It should be no surprise, then, that according to a study in *Social Psychology Quarterly,* if you can hang in with the same partner for twenty-five to thirty-five years, chances are that you and your mate will be very happy again, perhaps even as happy as you were as newlyweds. This study claims that following the honeymoon period in a marriage, a length of rope the study assumes lasts about four to five years, most relationships go through increasingly rocky times as a result of the familial responsibilities that absorb so much of our time, energy, spirit, and money, while also giving us so much of our satisfaction. After twenty-five years, however, this study claims, relationships start to improve because there are fewer parental and work responsibilities, as well as "an increase in assets," although judging from my own situation, I'm not sure how much you can count on an increase in your assets as you boom into your fifties. You can, however, count on the shrinking of your responsibilities just as soon as your kids are out the door. Even better, when the kids are finally gone, many parents establish even stronger ties with their newly adult offspring, ties based on mutual respect sans discipline. On the parents' side, the respect stems from the relief that their kids turned out all right after all. On the kids' side, the respect comes from their realization that Dad wasn't really as dumb as he seemed all those years. (I'm still waiting for my sons to tell me that, by the way, but hey, even my eldest has only been away from home for nine years.)

In middle age we often establish better relationships with our parents as well, in part because we become afraid that our parents are going to die before we make our peace with them (everyone has at least one issue with their parents, some of us way, way more than one), and on their side, our parents are usually finally willing to accept that we are not going to change much anymore. My mother, for example, has accepted that I am never going to become a specialist, so she has taken to calling me a "personality" instead, which isn't quite as good as say, an allergist or a dermatologist, but it is certainly better in the Florida Jewish women's pecking order than being "just a GP." And that has made a big difference in our relationship, although she still doesn't accept any medical advice from me. ("What do you know, Arthur? You're just a personality." See what I mean about issues?)

Then we come to our kids' kids. For some men (and I count myself among them), around fifty is when they first begin to realize that in the not-too-distant future they may become grandparents and they begin to look forward to preventing all those imperfections that, despite their undoubted parenting skills, marred their own kids. This happy expectation is even stronger now that I'm nearing the age of sixty than it was at fifty. In fact, I am so dying to become a granddad that every time I see her, I remind my beautiful, wonderful, brilliant, talented, sensitive daughter-in-law (and my son, too) that although they may have all the time in the world, my biological clock is tick, tick, ticking ever more forcefully, although so far, no luck, I'm afraid.

Anyway, the bottom line is that most family relationships and marriages, like fine wines and cheese, smell better with age.

But what about work? Surely, some of you would say, work can't possibly smell better at fifty. Or rather, surely, work smells to high heaven at fifty. And indeed, it often does. Thus, one of the most significant changes for midlife men is how we view, and are viewed in, our working lives. Most men define themselves to a great extent by the kind of achievers or providers they are, so young men are not so much what they eat as what they do, and in our formative adult years, we revel in the prospect of being the best ever at whatever we have chosen to do.

By our late forties, however, and sometimes well before that, most of us have stopped dreaming about becoming the CEO, the head announcer, the judge, the dean, the foreman, even the dominant con on the cell block, because by then we have grudgingly accepted that we have climbed about as high as we are going to climb in our particular job or calling or prison unit. By the age of fifty, most men are aware that even if we were to attempt to scale them, there are few occupational or vocational mountains available for us to climb, since base camps on those mountains are reserved for younger folk. But the curious thing is that, for many men, the realization that this is just about it, that we are now nearly out from under the canopy of gradually expanding expectations, comes as a great relief and allows us to look elsewhere—to the community or to our families, or even inwards—for new challenges and rewards. Thus, a recent study found that the happiest and hardest-working volunteers in community organizations were people in later midlife, and these were also the people who seemed to get the most psychological satisfaction out of volunteer work.

Also, by fifty, most men have stopped trying to compete in the game immortalized, as all great ideas are these days, in a bumper sticker that reads something like: "The guy with the most toys in the end wins." Happily, many of us have achieved a certain measure of comfort by our fifties, and we have probably bought nearly every contraption, gadget, and objet d'art that we or our partners would ever want to buy, and certainly we have most of the things we absolutely need, except, perhaps, for a leather toilet seat (actually, recently got that) and a sterling silver grape slicer (that, too). This realization also provides many men with a great sense of relief. I mean, you can't begin to imagine how much less stress I've had in my life since my wife conceded that the last renovation we did on the kitchen was probably the last kitchen renovation I would ever have to live through. Our contractor, however, was devastated. After all, how is he going to pay for his next Jaguar?

Most men also get much comfort when they hit fifty from finally admitting to themselves and to their mates that those unrealistic dreams they postponed "for a while, you know, just so I can get ahead with my job," will never actually be realized. This necessary insight allows us to finally stop dreaming and to concentrate on real life instead of reel life. I, for example, have now accepted that I will never learn to like herbal tea (I clearly aimed low in some of my goals), I will never play for the Montreal Canadiens (ditto), and I will never win the Nobel Prize. Well, not for peace, anyway. Literature? That's still open, I think. The obscure Polish poet and the pompous English playwright categories are already filled, but the whining Canadian Jewish male (there's only Cohen and moi, as far as I can see) category is not, so hey, I've got a shot.

Another benefit of becoming middle-aged is that we can now admit that the world is not as simple and that some of the good guys are not nearly as good as we'd always maintained but had long privately doubted. Thus, we can finally acknowledge that those left-wing politicians we used to support in our younger years often turned out to be even more arrogant and greedy and incompetent and self-serving than the other guys, just as our dads predicted. So, it's OK to admit that to ourselves now and to vote for the other guys, although we may not want to reveal it to our friends. For most midlife men who come from a liberal background, comme moi, it also comes as a great relief to be able to hand over responsibility for whales, dolphins, rain forests, animal experimentation, ozone, tobacco, fish farms, and so on to a younger generation, whose members don't yet have lawns, mortgages, hemorrhoids, and retirement funds to worry about.

In short, a fifty-year-old man has finally grown up, and he takes a lot of satisfaction from the successes he has achieved and the relationships he has fostered.

Man Looking Down

But all is not always as rosy as I've painted it, of course, especially for those midlifers who, like me, are nearing sixty, because the older we get, the more we suffer from some other kinds of burdens that are not loaded onto the shoulders of younger dudes. One of the increasingly important concerns for many midlifers is the issue of parenting—backwards, because taking care of our kids has been replaced by having to take care of our parents. The happy news, though, is that not only do most of us seem to handle this burden with our usual aplomb but also many aged parents are still quite independent, thank God, many defiantly so.

A perfect example of that previous optimistic assessment is my relationship with my mom, who specifically asked to be mentioned more in this edition of *Midlife Man* than she was in the first one. ("You're not proud of your mother, Arthur? What do you mean, the book is not about me? You're about me, so everything you write is about me." Go argue with that, I told my editor.) Much to my surprise, not to mention that of everyone who knows me, my mom and I have actually grown closer in the last couple of years. The reason for our new-found closeness is straightforward: my mom needs me now and I thrive on being needed.

My mom has, not surprisingly, grown more frail the last few years (although as she never ceases to point out, everyone says she looks much younger than her stated age), but much more surprisingly, my mom has grown more insecure, too. The frailty has been relatively easy to deal with, since on my part it has involved little beyond offers to help my mom with her shopping, driving her to appointments, and doing odd jobs around her house (the jobs have to be very, very odd for me to be able to do them).

The psychological changes, however, have been much more difficult to accept and deal with. My mom, after all, is a Holocaust survivor, a woman who always prided herself on her abilities to take care of everything that needed taking care of, a woman who used to say, with fierce emphasis, "If Hitler didn't get me, Arthur, nothing will." And she meant it.

But now she is unsure of many little things that she used to do without hesitation, and for which she asks my help. She also now regularly calls to ask for my advice, something she had done occasionally before, but these days she actually listens to what I have to say. My mom still manages all her financial affairs herself and she still knows to the penny what's due her or what she owes (not that she ever owes anyone even a penny, another remnant of surviving the Holocaust), but she needs constant help with decisions, with choices, with the kinds of problems we all solve for ourselves without much thought or anxiety.

So all that has driven us to be much closer. In fact, last year, my mom even abandoned her beloved Montreal ("It's the most beautiful city in the world, Arthur." "Not if you have to live there, Ma.") and moved to Vancouver to be with my wife and me, and what has been eye-popping to me is that this new proximity has resulted in a huge improvement in our relationship because we have developed a much greater mutual respect. On my part, I have been amazed at my mom's ability to cope with the many changes that have been forced on her. First she had to decide to leave Montreal and the place my father is buried (until she came out west, my mom used to visit my father's grave every week to talk to him and keep him up-to-date on the family); then she had to buy a new home in Vancouver and sell the house she had lived in for forty years; and finally, she had to pack up all her belongings, say goodbye to her remaining friends, many of whom are quite ill, and relocate out here. This would be a hard haul for a person in their twenties with a helping partner. My mom is over eighty (I don't know how much over eighty because she won't tell me) and alone. Yet she did it all by herself with only minimal help from her oldest son and his amazingly patient and helpful wife. But here's the thing: as I write this, she is thriving in her new environment, all of which has awed me with her abilities.

Happily, I think my mom has gained a lot of respect for me, too. Now, my mom has always unashamedly bragged about me to anyone silly enough to ask: "My son, the doctor," and "My son on TV," and "My son, the personality," and much more. But, to be frank, I never believed she thought much of my abilities because, as I wrote earlier, she has never really had occasion to use my help, and when she did ask for my advice she never took it.

That has all changed now. I have to help my mom with a lot of little things and I think she has finally understood that I will come through for her, something that, because of our strained relationship, she may not have completely believed before. Thus, she has trusted my wife and me to help her with the move out west, although despite her protestations that "You're in charge, Arthur, and I'll do everything you say," she still managed to slip a ton of stuff that I had tried to throw out into the moving crates (my mom is the only person in Canada, I am sure, to have shipped six rolls of paper towels across the country at an astounding cost per roll merely because she had bought them at a bargain price and couldn't bear to throw them out).

I know that this new-found respect between the two of us may yet founder, especially if my mom begins to evince any signs of mental deterioration, which, thank God, she has not shown yet. But for now, the happy news is that contrary to what I expected, the relationship between this midlife man and his aged P is thriving. And I am certain the same applies to many other guys in my situation.

Another area of concern for many aging midlife men is the effect that volatile economic conditions might have on their lives, especially on their jobs. In many industries and professions, a fifty-year-old middle-class man has become an expendable commodity. And if you haven't been a good saver, fifty can seem very close to sixty-five, and sixty is even closer.

That said, it's been very interesting for me to observe how many of my friends have walked away from work between the ages of fifty and sixty—those that could afford to walk away from their jobs, of course. Thus, all of my several closest friends (I know the idea of having "several closest friends" makes me sound an awful lot like a teenage girl, but I do, in fact, have several closest friends) have either cut their work hours back significantly or have taken buyout packages or sold their businesses. And as I had predicted, most of them have turned to community work to take up much of their now spare time (well, it's either that or divorce since their wives sure don't want them hanging around the house any more than is absolutely necessary). And they seem very content with their new roles in life.

Another area of concern for some guys at this age is "our looks" because midlife is when most of us discover that we no longer matter as much or at all to "chicks." As a man I know who claims he has bedded many women and who still looks about ten years younger than his real age of fifty five put it to me one day, "It's really scary, man, because the young, good-looking chicks just don't look at me any longer." Although I could understand his lament—the good-looking chicks haven't looked at me for many years, if they ever did—I could not really understand his panic (or the reason he still talks like a teenager). After all, why should a young woman, who has to be careful about the quality of the DNA she accepts into that single egg she will deliver that month, want to be impregnated by an older and perhaps less healthy specimen, when she can have her pick of younger and more desirable DNA?

Happily, though, most middle-aged men accept this change in our sexual status, albeit somewhat ruefully, and we generally go gentle into the next stage of our sexual maturity. (An old joke: A man of a certain age is accosted by a younger attractive woman who whispers an offer into his ear. "Super sex." "I'll take the soup," he replies instantly.) Some middle-aged men, however, are overwhelmed by this disappearing interest from the younger members of the other side, which partially explains why a disproportionate number of these guys seek out a trophy wife (or if they're Hollywood stars—such as Michael Douglas, Robert Redford, Harrison Ford, or Jack Nicholson—a young chicklet to bed and/or co-star with) to give the world the metaphoric finger and to let everyone know that "Hey! I'm still as desirable as I ever was. Just look at this woman on my arm. She proves that the chicks still dig me." The only problem is that this guy has to wake up every morning next to someone who, when he tells her that the day Kennedy died is still perhaps the most meaningful and formative moment in his life, can't figure out why this geezer next to her would get so worked up about that guy they made fun of on *Seinfeld* and who died in that plane accident.

Of far more concern to most older midlife men are the first intimations of mortality that most of us feel around fifty, a time when we start to worry about getting sick, and when we begin to chart the various problems—diabetes, osteoporosis, heart attacks, arthritis—that our friends have come down with. Worse, this is also the time of life when we realize that death is not as far off as we had always thought it to be, and why, oh why, didn't we listen to our father and buy more life insurance. This fear is usually hammered home to us by news of someone our age who is either very sick or who may even have died. "Did you hear about Brian? Keeled over. Right in the middle of the deli. I never trusted those pickles, you know. What do you mean his doctor said the pickles had nothing to do with it? What do those doctors know anyway?" As an aside, I must shamefacedly admit that despite the fact that I used to make constant fun of my mother-in-law for this habit, I too now read the obits every day (although contrary to what one of my friends claims, I don't shout "Beat another one" when I recognize a familiar name in the list).

So given many men's concerns about their health and mortality, it's no surprise that fifty is also the age of alarm, and many midlife men respond to these worries by suddenly determining to do all those healthy lifestyle things they should have been doing all along. Take me, for example. Because of a sort of panic response (I freaked about my weight, not my mortality), I took up an exercise regimen about seven years ago, which has, surprisingly, turned out to be one of the best decisions of my life, and to know why you will have to read Chapter 7 (but finish this one first).

Finally, there are the guys who probably take the arrival of midlife the hardest: those middle-aged men who have attained a great deal of power—and after all, despite their bleating, middle-aged guys are still by and large the ones who run the world. Such men tend to see midlife changes as a real threat not only to their status but to their entire sense of self. To these guys, the physical changes of midlife—the belly, the wrinkles, the thinning hair, the fatigue, as well as the evident disdain, or worse, lack of attention, from younger folks—represent weakness, vulnerability, the passing of their king-of-the-hill potency, blood to the hordes of younger people baying at their heels. To a large extent, I think, these are the guys who are flocking to doctors, desperate to find a solution, preferably a hormonal or chemical one, to temporarily derail the inevitable by reversing any signs of aging and by allaying any symptoms they have, especially those that stand as public indications of their declining youthful vigour (some symptoms don't stand of course; in fact, the problem is just the opposite). These are the men so desperate to stay young and powerful forever that they will do anything, believe anything, that tells them they are not as old as the calendar says they are.

The Way It Is

So that's how guys are at middle age. Some are threatened, a few are devastated, but most are happy and satisfied—at least as happy as they are ever going to be. And that is why I take issue with those New Age authors and gurus who are trying to convince middle-aged guys that they are not really as happy as they think, that they need more purpose in life, and that they should be busily preparing for the next phase, in which they will become mentors and purveyors of wisdom to the younger men following behind them. Well, I've got news for those know-nothing drummers in the mud: that message is, to quote my sagacious son, "a load of crap" (that boy is going to leave his mark somewhere; I just hope it's not at home). First, we're not unhappy. Most of us are doing all right, Jack. Second, we're still busy, and have no time to mentor. Most important, though, the men behind us are no different from what we were like at their age, and they don't want to hear from us, just as I never wanted to hear my father's advice until it was too late to benefit from it. I used to cringe and even leave the room when my dad used the word "experience" in his effort to teach me something, mostly because I never wanted to experience what he had endured ("Experience," said Oscar Wilde, "is the name every one gives to their mistakes"), and with typical youthful arrogance I was equally certain that he had never experienced what I was going through. Things are no different today, of course. In what I can only think of as appropriate retribution, my sons cringe whenever I insert that terrifying phrase "when I was your age" into anything I tell them. Worse, though, rather than leave the room, they begin to laugh at me, at which point I usually leave the room.

Despite the wailing of the men-who-drum, the truth is that the men and boys behind us don't want our insight, our accumulated wisdom, the knowledge we have gleaned from hard experience. They just want us outta here ASAP so that they can take over sooner.

And so it should be. Middle age is not a preparatory stage for mentoring but should be enjoyed for itself. What we must do is revel in our moment as members of the happiest demographic group around and from this self-satisfied perch build on what we have so that we are better able to handle the inevitable trials of old age.

I'll close this section by quoting the words of Ronald Kessler, a sociologist at MIDMAC (cited by Winifred Gallagher in *Atlantic Monthly*), who has said, "the data show that middle age is the very best time in life." In fact, "the best year is fifty." Why? Because, says Kessler, "you don't have to deal with the aches and pains of old age or the anxieties of youth... You're healthy. You're productive. You have enough money to do some of the things you like to do. You've come to terms with your relationships, and the chance of divorce is very low. Midlife is the 'it' you've been working toward." And happily, for most of us, this is still very largely true nearing sixty, too.

{2}

WHY DO I LOOK AND FEEL THE WAY I DO?

• • •

It's not the men in my life, it's the life in my men.

MAE WEST, *I'm No Angel*

So believe it or not, fifty is the "it" you have relentlessly been marching towards all those formative years. That's the good news. The inevitable bad news, however, is that "it" is not quite nirvana because "it" is often accompanied by some unwelcome physical alterations.

Before I move on to discuss those changes, however, I have to offer a disclaimer. For those of you who have been lured into buying this book by reading the dust jacket, which implies that a disproportionate amount of the text is devoted to sexual matters and sexual parts, my deep apologies. To be sure, that is certainly what my publisher wanted. "Sex sells," he pointedly mentioned, even before I had written the first paragraph. Indeed, every time he called me to discuss the project, he invariably whined something like, "Couldn't you put just a bit more sex into it, Art? At the very least, can't you move the sex parts up to the front where they belong?"

In this focus on sex, my publisher was merely reflecting the common misconception that if sex is not the only health issue that matters to men—young, middle-aged, and old—it is certainly the most important one, a belief seemingly borne out in the last few years by the frenzy over erectile dysfunction drugs. Now I suppose this view that "sex is all that matters" is true for some men, but even penis-driven ever-ready automatons who just keep coming and coming and coming usually realize as they begin to age that man cannot live by bed alone, which is why, I strongly believe, most men are just as interested in and concerned about the changes that occur to their other body parts and functions. I will concede, however, that sex is very important, and so it has been given its own chapter (Chapter 3). For now we will concentrate on all those other changes that happen to your body as you hit your middle years.

Peau, Peau Me

For a startling example of the difference between your middle-aged skin and the skin of a younger person, here's an easy experiment you can try. First, after obtaining permission, of course, gently pinch a younger person's skin, preferably in a sun-exposed area. See how quickly it snaps back into place? Now pinch your own skin and watch as it slowly sinks back to a semblance of flatness. See how long it takes? Your skin has begun to dry out; hers has not yet started to.

In middle age, skin has begun to sag and desiccate and bunch up and wrinkle and prune. It also becomes less elastic and more mottled, and you begin to notice an increasing number of those small blood vessels that are a sure giveaway of aging skin. And as we all know from pictures of Bob Dylan and Keith Richards, man, these normal components of aging are greatly accentuated by accumulated damage from excess exposure to the sun and from poor lifestyle habits, especially smoking. ("So what exactly was it that was blowin' in the wind in those sixties, Dad?" my son recently smirked. Tell me again why it is we have children.) Not surprisingly, these changes can be very disturbing to some people. For example, a survey done for Ortho Pharmaceuticals found that wrinkles disturb boomers more than grey hair does, in part, I suppose, because so many middle-aged guys no longer have enough hair to be concerned about its colour, although they certainly have lots of wrinkles to worry about. To minimize these changes, stay out of the sun as much as possible and just peacefully accept that your time as a bronzed sun god has come and most assuredly gone. Or as my son would say, "cover up, dude." And don't smoke anything, of course.

As to treatment, a growing number of my peers have begun to visit plastic surgeons—excuse me, cosmetic surgeons—although according to the American Academy of Cosmetic Surgery, women still dominate the cosmetic surgery market by a wide margin, and at all ages. To serve the increasing number of middle-aged men who want to enhance what nature bestowed on them, cosmetic surgeons now offer a rapidly increasing cornucopia of choices—botulism toxin injections, collagen injections, chemical peels, laser procedures, nose jobs, dermabrasion, liposuction, face-lifts, a ton of new products to inject into the skin and deeper tissues, all types of surgical "enhancements," and all manner of inserts that can alter any outward part of you in ways your mother never thought possible. ("What's the matter with looking like your father, Arthur? He was a very handsome man." Memory is a funny thing, eh?) If you have the money and the inclination, then by all means do what my wife makes me do to the furniture regularly and rearrange. It's your life, after all, and you should look any way you like, although if all you're seeking is the right form for wearing a Speedo, don't do it. The rule is simple: no man is allowed in public wearing a Speedo.

There is also a host of skin care products you can use, such as alpha hydroxy acid creams or tretinoin, a derivative of vitamin A, to hide the effects of aging and ultraviolet radiation damage. And they do work to improve wrinkling, surface roughness, and even some of the colour changes that occur in photo-damaged skin. If you ask me, though, a real man would never resort to such artifice, and besides, when I used it, the tretinoin was very irritating.

The Hair Apparent

As we age, our hair begins to lose colour and turn grey because of a fall in the number of active melanocytes, the cells that govern skin and hair pigment. No wonder, then, that a recent survey found one-third of men are using some sort of hair dye, even though the jury is still out on whether these dyes increase the risk of some cancers.

But it's not just more grey hair that we suffer with the years. With increasing age, the number of hair follicles on our scalps decreases, and the rate of growth of the hair in the still active follicles also slows, often to a metaphoric crawl. Take me, for example. I once required a haircut every three weeks; I now get my hair attended to only once every six weeks, and even then my stylist (she used to be my barber back when I used to be her doctor, not her health care provider) spends more time trimming my wallet than the back of my scalp. In God's great joke, however, while hair on our scalps becomes thinner and sparser in middle age, hair on other parts of our bodies starts to grow, even to blossom, which is why most middle-aged guys have to regularly and painfully extract hair from various openings in their skulls. Who knew that hair could grow in so many difficult-to-access places? And so fast, too.

Hair loss in young and middle-aged men, which is now thought to be largely inherited from the mother (thanks a lot, Ma), although the father's genes clearly play a role, too, is a lot more common than you may think. Twenty per cent of men start to lose hair by age twenty-five, and in a recent study, researchers concluded that by middle age, 50 per cent of men have some of what they call MPHL, which sounds more like a hockey league than what it really stands for—male-pattern hair loss. This study also found, as you would expect, that men make more of a to-do about their do than neutral observers, in large part, of course, because for a balding man his hair loss is an embarrassingly public signal of growing old. No surprise, then, that North American men (and increasingly women, too) spend billions of dollars on hair-growth therapies every year.

So what have I done about my hair loss, you are no doubt wondering if you have seen my picture on the dust jacket. To be honest, I twice tried to do something about it. First, as a much younger man, on the advice of my hirsute barber, whose name was something like Pappa Doc (I think he was a Rastafarian—he always wore one of those caps, and there was always an interesting smell in the shop, which is mostly why I kept going back—every few days), I purchased some mustard oil and diligently applied it to my scalp for several weeks. Although Pappa Doc had assured me that the mustard oil would slow my hair loss, it didn't, although it did cause my scalp to burn and make me smell terrible. For some worrisome reason, though, no one seemed to treat me any differently.

The second therapy I tried was Rogaine, or topical minoxidil, a shampoo that works somewhat for a small proportion of men, although it clearly did nothing for me. That's when I gave up so I never tried the drug finasteride, which is used to treat benign prostatic hyperplasia (see Chapter 4) and is also much promoted as a hair-growth stimulant under the name Propecia. Studies show that both Rogaine and Propecia can produce modest increases in hair growth, but you had better have deep pockets to go with your shiny scalp because the minute you discontinue these drugs, you start losing hair again. Furthermore, although these products have been available for over ten years now, and the safety record thus far is a good one, we still don't fully know what the long-term consequences of using them for many years might be (such as, for example, hairy palms from applying the shampoo regularly). The other thing that stopped me from using Propecia is that the list of potential side effects includes loss of libido and erectile dysfunction, and if you ask me, there is probably nothing more frustrating than to be well coifed but with no interest or ability to go where your hair is itching to take you.

After these two self-administered treatments, you are left with rugs and slugs and thugs: the first referring to hairpieces, of course, the second being my term for the always cautious and slow cosmetic surgeons who make fortunes off the various procedures required to make your scalp look like, well, a scalp that has had hair transplanted onto it, and the third referring to those people who separate you from your hard-earned money by sticking a type of laser on your skull that is supposed to restore lost hair, but which, according to most doctors, does absolutely nothing except fatten the wallets of the laser owners.

If all that's not for you, though, two exciting possibilities on the horizon are gene therapy and a sort of hair follicle cloning, what the people working on it are calling follicular neogenesis, although if you're middle-aged I wouldn't hold my breath waiting for either of these to hit the market soon enough to matter for you. Your male heirs' hairs might benefit from them, however.

Finally, if you ask me, the best thing to do about a thinning or even totally slimmed scalp is the same as I would advise for changes in the skin: just grin and bare it. There is a rather pleasant compensation to baldness, you see, and that is that many people equate lack of hair on the scalp with extra brain matter in the cranium. And this has long been the case. For example, according to Shakespeare, a man who started the science of psychology, after all, "There's many a man has more hair than wit," although some would probably say that the prematurely balding playwright had a distinct conflict of interest when it came to matters of the scalp. But as always, the Bard, who never heard something in the street he couldn't use, was merely reflecting popular sentiment that is current even today. For example, according to a study from Denison University in Ohio, both men and women claimed that bald men in the pictures they looked at were smarter than their more hirsute brothers.

More Fat on Thinning Bones

Perhaps the most depressing study I came across in my research is one that concluded that unless a middle-aged man continually increases the number of calories he burns every day, he will inevitably get fatter by roughly ten pounds a decade (this exact number has recently been called into question but the overall conclusion has not been challenged), a finding easily verified by perusing any typical gathering, where so many middle-aged guys look as if they're auditioning to become Michelin Man stand-ins. Middle-aged men also begin to lose muscle mass. How much muscle is lost? Lots. Starting at about the sixth decade of life, according to one estimate, people lose about 10 to 12 per cent of muscle strength and 6 per cent of muscle mass per decade on average.

As well, our bones begin to thin slowly from early adulthood, a process that accelerates rapidly in midlife. Unhappily, too, degenerative arthritis (see Chapter 5) is becoming much more common in midlife, especially in those baby boomers who spent so many of their young adult years running with far too much intensity and for far too many miles on hard surfaces (Remember when it was "no pain, no gain"? Boy were we ever wrong!) and who have now come down with degenerative arthritis in their hips and/or knees, which in many cases, unfortunately, has resulted in the need for hip or knee replacement surgery. That said, all middle-aged men, athletes or not, complain of more aches and pains than they did when younger, and they also find that it takes longer to recover from nagging soft tissue injuries such as muscle pulls. This is all a reflection of increasingly inelastic ligaments and tendons, as well as less springy articular cartilage, the tissues that provide cushioning in the joints.

Exercise and a healthy diet (discussed in Chapters 6 and 7) can, of course, somewhat slow these tendencies, although they are relentlessly inevitable, alas.

Losing Your Senses

The lens of the eye starts to thicken in middle age, leading to poorer night vision and poorer ability to focus, especially for close objects, which explains, of course, why many middle-agers need to work so hard to find the best distance to hold a page from their noses, and why so many middle-aged men stare so hard at beautiful young women. It's not that they're leering; it's just that they can't see them well enough.

What happens to our hearing faculties as we age is best illustrated in this old story in which a middle-aged man tells a friend, "You know, my wife left me." "Why?" asks the friend. "Because she says I never listen to her. At least that's what I think she said."

It's true. Like the sense of vision, the sense of hearing also diminishes in middle age, more rapidly in men than in women, and especially for higher tones. (You think that has anything to do with the fact that women's voices are so high in tone? Nahh, couldn't be.)

Although sense of taste and smell are commonly said to get worse with age, it's still unclear how rapidly these losses take hold. On the one hand, a report from Duke University claims that loss of taste and smell are common as we age. On the ever-present other hand, a study from the Claude Pepper Center for Research on Oral Health at the University of Florida found that in some people the senses of touch, taste, and smell deteriorate only slightly with age, but that they deteriorate much more rapidly in people who smoke or drink too much alcohol. So don't do that. Next.

Taking Your Breath Away, Then Breaking Your Heart

The respiratory system becomes less efficient in middle age because the lungs start to lose some of their essential elasticity, resulting in poorer oxygenation of the blood. If you're still stupid enough to be smoking in midlife, middle age is when you generally begin to notice the first signs of chronic bronchitis or emphysema—chronic, persistent cough, increasing shortness of breath, and mucus production—and middle age is certainly when you will first begin to worry that you might have lung cancer, a fear that, like Britney Spears and Madonna videos, will return to haunt you with increasing and sickening regularity.

In middle age, our hearts also become less efficient and potentially more erratic, resulting in increasing risks of heart rhythm abnormalities such as atrial fibrillation. For many of us in midlife, our heart rate can't go up as rapidly during exercise as it once did and aerobic capacity begins to fall. The former is actually a very important prognostic sign about the state of your arteries. Thus, according to a French study, how much your heart rate goes up with exercise and how quickly after exercise your heart rate returns to normal are key indicators of how likely you are to die prematurely of a sudden heart attack. So what numbers are we looking at? In this study, middle-aged men (all French civil service workers, meaning that they weren't exactly killing themselves at work; the French have perfected the four-day weekend, which happens every weekend during the summer) whose heart rates didn't speed up to at least 89 beats per minute or whose heart rates didn't slow down by at least 25 beats per minute after exercise had a significantly higher risk of dying from a sudden heart attack over the subsequent decade than did men whose heart rates did speed up to more than 89 beats per minute or whose hearts slowed by 25 beats per minute. And men whose resting heart rate was over 75 had a higher risk of sudden death than men whose resting heart rate was less than 75, thus emphasizing the observation that the resting heart rate is really a lot like limbo (the West Indian dance—not the place Catholics might go): the lower, the better, so that 80 beats per minute may be fine, but 60 is better. So just what is your resting heart rate and how much does it speed up when you run?

In midlife, our arteries have already become significantly less elastic and continue to get worse in those of us who don't live a healthy lifestyle (sadly, this defect of less elastic arteries is now showing up in rapidly increasing numbers of young kids, too, because so many kids are fat and sedentary, and that's something that bodes very poorly for their futures since elasticity is an important feature of healthy arteries). Also, in our middle years, the one-way valves in our veins stop being as efficient as they once were, which is why so many of us start developing varicose veins.

As usual, not smoking, doing enough exercise (Chapter 7), and maintaining a healthy weight are the keys to minimizing the effects from these changes.

Urine in Big Trouble, Boy

The kidneys shrink as we get older, and their filtering efficiency also begins to fall. For me, one of the worst things about middle age has been the fact that, well, I just can't hold it as well as I used to, although to be honest, I never held it very well because to compensate for our huge brains and great looks, God clearly balanced the books by burdening Hister men with small bladders. But as we age not only does the bladder begin to develop less capacity to store urine, it also doesn't empty itself as well when you direct it to unload, which is why, dear readers, for me, as for so many guys who don't plan well and drink a double cappuccino before entering the cinema, there is at least one one-minute gap in every movie, sometimes two or three. I still don't know, for example, why that Jeremy Irons and his Italian crowd hated Shylock so much. Was it Al Pacino's accent? His overacting?

There are also the inevitable changes associated with prostate enlargement (see Chapter 4), which occur in every man who lives long enough and can lead to difficulty starting the urinary stream. (Ever stand next to a seventy-year-old at a bank of urinals and watch how long it takes him to get his business done? Well, you really shouldn't watch—just stare straight ahead and count silently, but bear in mind that it will be a very long count.) Prostate enlargement can also lead to difficulty stopping, urgency, which is defined as the need to go—NOW, leaking (hiding those yellow stains is the most important reason to lower the toilet seat after use, my wife unkindly says), and the need to get up at night to urinate.

Falling Energy Reserves

In middle age, our energy levels fall to varying degrees. Thus, some midlife guys complain that they just don't have enough energy to get around or do some of the things they used to do as vim-filled young bucks—male-defining activities such as bear hunting and beer pong—while other guys don't complain about falling energy levels at all. They just go to bed at nine P.M., two hours after their wives hit the sack. No matter how we handle it, though, this energy drop is, alas, universal in midlife, as anyone who has ever been stuck in a room full of middle-aged yawners at nine P.M. can attest.

Middle-agers also sleep differently than younger men. Not only do we go to bed sooner, we also can't fall asleep as easily as we once did, we sleep less deeply than we used to, our sleep is not as efficient as it was when we were younger so we rise feeling less rested after a night's sleep, and according to a British study in *Occupational and Environmental Medicine,* people in midlife also tend to rise earlier than younger people do and to fade sooner "after lunch"; I for one believe that completely, because these days, I often fade before lunch.

The good news is that there are a host of strategies to help you sleep better (see Chapter 7).

Fading Mental Abilities

Although men start out with more brain cells than women (not surprising since young men need those bigger brains to remember all those vital sports statistics and data on cars and video game comparisons that they retain so well), men also lose brain cells three times as fast as women as they age. Thus, by age forty-five, men's brains and women's brains are roughly the same size, although egos, most women would insist, continue to remain much larger in men, a claim that can actually be supported by a study that found that although men are much more confident than women that they can remember where they left the car keys, women are actually much better than men at knowing where misplaced items might be found. Although the loss of any brain cells is a problem, the loss of brain cells with age is unfortunately most acute in the frontal lobes, those areas that govern cognitive functions such as mental flexibility and attention span, a finding that might explain aging men's obsession with channel surfing and our inability to recall anything our wives thought we should have overheard and retained—but we didn't—at a cocktail party. Brain cells are also lost in the hippocampus and midbrain, a diminution of brain matter that affects memory and the sense of time elapsed from a given moment. Thus, time really does seem to be catching up to you much more quickly the older you get.

But why, you may well wonder as you are busily flipping channels and not finding anything that can keep your attention for more than a millisecond, do men lose more brain cells than women do? My wife's theory is that God figured that men wouldn't miss their brain cells as much as women would, but there's no real proof of that. According to a more objective theory, we men are just not able to switch off our brains, while women can easily put their brains into neutral, an observation that any man who has ever listened to a group of women chatting will no doubt instantly affirm. According to this theory, men, however, may not be easily able to let go of thinking furiously about something, anything, even while at rest. This is not really surprising when you consider all the important things constantly on our minds—when it's safe enough to ask for a break from painting so we can nap, whether our team can beat the points spread, whether to put mustard on before the ketchup, and so on. Consequently, this theory claims, men suffer the equivalent of an overuse injury of the brain; they may "burn out" some parts of their brains more quickly than women.

Fortunately, there are some things you can do to arrest this process, including getting lots of exercise and staying mentally active (see Chapter 7).

If That's Life, Do I Ever Need Help

So there you have it, guys—some of the important changes that will happen to you as you proceed through your midlife passage, although as I have pointed out frequently, you can at least slow down some of these changes (and even postpone many of them) by adopting some good lifestyle habits, as described in Chapters 6 and 7.

No matter how hard you try to avoid them, though, you must always accept that many (perhaps all?) of these changes will gradually hit you anyway. That's just the way it goes, I'm afraid, when you get older. Time exacts a toll.

That said, you might take at least some consolation from this: turning fifty certainly beats—by a wide margin—the only current known alternative to not turning fifty. You're welcome.

{3}

SEX AND THE MIDDLE-AGED MALE

• • •

The emphasis on performance is the
single greatest enemy of a satisfactory sexual life.
GAIL SHEEHY, "The Unspeakable Passage," *Vanity Fair*

Leonard Cohen, a man who's clearly been there and certainly done that (when I come back, I hope it's as a black-garbed, smoky-voiced poet), has complained in song that he aches in places where he used to play. Although most of us have not been fortunate enough to play nearly as hard and as often as Leonard has and certainly not on the same squad that Leonard managed to be drafted for, the reality is that even if we were always just subs and never made it onto the first-string team, most middle-aged guys are, like Leonard, aching in places that once used to be ache-free.

Now before you leap to a fallacious conclusion, let me quickly interpose that I'm absolutely certain that Leonard was using "ache" in a metaphorical sense. In other words, it's not so much that middle-aged guys experience physical pain in the old playground; it's more that our seesaw doesn't go as high as it used to when we were younger. Some guys are even finding that they cannot get their seesaw off the ground any longer, the countervailing weight, either emotional or physical, having become too heavy to be lifted without appropriate assistance. And that is why, of course, Viagra and its clones have become this era's hula hoops and pet rocks. Or as Julius Caesar would say now, "Vini, vidi, Viagra."

Sexual Changes in Midlife—Good to the Last Droop

What does happen to sexual functioning in middle age in men? Not much, really, but way too much. For a start, a man's testicles shrink slightly as he ages (and in case you're interested in seeing how you measure up, I don't know anyone who has actually had his measured, nor do I know of any health plan that would pay for this procedure, nor for that matter, do I know any health professionals who admit to doing this for a living). Testicles also don't ride as high as they used to, the aging male's scrotum tends not to shrink as much when he becomes aroused (shrinkage does not just happen to length of appendage, please note), and the number of testosterone-producing cells begins to drop. And while we're on the topic of testicles, this is a good place to mention that you should do a testicular self examination, or TSE, regularly. ("What do I do?" I hear some of you lesser lights asking. Easy, man. All you gotta do is roll your own.)

Other changes to sexual functioning include:

- a smaller volume of pre-ejaculatory secretions
- reduced sperm production and semen volume
- a small drop-off in the percentage of mature sperm that are most capable of fertilizing an anxious yet hopeful ovum

Overall, most middle-aged men still produce enough sperm to be able to impregnate a partner, if not quite on demand, then at least with effort, in time ("With effort, in time," by the way, is the old Hister family motto), although a recent study has concluded that achieving those pregnancies represents quite a trick for the average older guy because the rate of miscarriage goes up quite a bit with the increasing age of the father.

In addition, erections begin to change in midlife. Now I realize that many of you, especially the younger men reading this, might have trouble understanding that last bit. For most younger guys, after all, an erection is much like an elevator in a multi-storey building—it goes up and it goes down; the view while the elevator is in use is generally non-varying, and aside from the speed at which the elevator delivers you from the depths of the basement to the exhilaration of the penthouse, there really isn't much else to appreciate or criticize about it. And happily, that's usually the way it goes in the early years: up and down, up and down, on command, when in demand, zipping rapidly between floors to deliver its cargo to the luxurious upstairs suites, and requiring minimal maintenance, not even any regular lubrication. But even the most pampered and well-maintained elevator can sometimes get stuck between floors. It might even malfunction on occasion by lingering on lower-level floors. Worst of all, like HAL, the computer in *2001—A Space Odyssey,* some elevators seem to develop minds of their own and no matter how much attention is paid (to cite Arthur Miller about another Willy, one named Loman), they prefer to stay grounded most of the time, despite their handlers' best attempts to get them moving upwards into service. That's how it is with erections, too. During middle age, not only do many men begin to suffer from occasional bouts of erectile dysfunction, or ED, but even a midlife man who is always able (with effort, in time) to get hard enough to do his duty tends to suffer a bit of loss of upward mobility of his penis due to changes in the blood vessels that are responsible for creating and maintaining an erection. These changes also lead to a slight alteration in the angle of the erection.

Middle age also brings changes to the quality of a man's erection so that men at this age begin to complain of erections they describe as "softer" or "weaker." Not only, then, does it take most middle-aged guys longer to achieve even a garden-variety, run-of-the-mill erection, but in contrast to when they were young, when a rock-hard erection immediately sprang up after even the slightest erotic thought (prompted by a drop of water, for example, or a leaf wavering in the wind), in midlife, some men require direct hands-on contact, that is, physical stimulation, without which they are unable to hit full hardness, and even then, it's rarely as hard as they'd like it to be. How do we know all this? you ask. Because there are people out there who study these things, and they have actually developed a way of measuring the strength of erections, or at least what those erections are able to do, which is sort of the same thing. (Those of you reading this to your kids as a bedtime story might want to skip the next part.) In *Clock of Ages*, Dr. John Medina claims that "ejaculatory distance" drops off from "two feet in young men to only minimal dribbling distance in the elderly," and I'll bet that until you read that, you had absolutely no idea that they even held that kind of competition. Well, they clearly do, and I'm certain it's a sellout every time.

For some middle-aged men, even with physical stimulation there is often no there, there (to paraphrase Gertrude Stein's comment about Oakland). In other words, middle age is when increasing numbers of men begin to be visited by that unwelcome bedroom spectre known as ED, who is inevitably greeted like a death figure in a comedy/horror movie, come to call on the wrong guy at the wrong time. ("Oh, God, not now, not now. Can't you see I'm about to score?") For men who begin to be troubled by intermittent but increasingly frequent visits from this frightening apparition, a diamond-hard erection becomes elusive, and for a small but growing number of men, it becomes rarer to experience a trouble-free sexual episode than to discover a Hollywood dimbo who doesn't feel the need to author a series of children's books. And eventually (alas!) for a huge number of aged men, a usable erection is like Bigfoot: it clearly exists, but you know you'll never see one in your lifetime.

Midlife man also finds that his orgasm becomes shorter. "But how much shorter can it get?" asked my smirking wife, proving how little attention she actually pays to what I tell her. It's orgasm that they're talking about, not foreplay. With increasing age, a man's erection also detumesces faster—that is, his rocket plummets to earth more quickly than it did in the old days, and he can't relaunch nearly as rapidly for a second flight. "Second flight?" my wife chimed in here. "I'd just settle for a faster cab to the airport." You know, most of the time, I have no idea what that woman is talking about, and I don't think I want to know.

These generally gradual changes are, unfortunately, universal with advancing years, and no man is immune, but clearly they don't hit all men equally hard (or not, as the case may be). Furthermore, no matter how mild or severe the changes may be, men respond to them in very different ways. After all, the brain is still the biggest and certainly the most important sexual organ, so while some guys are devastated by even the slightest change in their sexual apparatus or functioning, others seem to absorb significant changes with only minimal complaints. And now that ED drugs are available, ever-growing numbers of midlife men are appearing in doctors' offices to get help stiffening their resolve.

Arise, You Prisoners of Deflation

Impotence—or as the experts now refer to it, erectile dysfunction—is the inability to obtain and sustain an erection for satisfactory intercourse, which leads inevitably to the questions, how do you define "satisfactory" and who is doing the defining?

Erectile dysfunction is a major concern for many—actually all—men. (And I must say it's a name I simply loathe because it reminds me of my kids' toy erector set and how my own constructions always kept falling over. "Maybe it's a lesson for later life," my wise wife used to say. See what I mean about having no clue what that woman is ever on about?) Thus, one American survey found that if given the choice, men would rather go deaf and blind and end up in severe pain than have their wan wee willie wilt—that is, a majority of men said they would rather have a hearing impairment, cataracts, high blood pressure, and arthritis than ED, although the great joke on these guys is that as typical North American men, they are likely to end up with all of the above, including ED, anyway.

The incidence of ED rises gradually with age (although men don't) and doubles every decade. According to a widely cited study, by age forty, 5 per cent of men are frequently unable to perform when called on, while more than 30 per cent report occasional difficulties performing. By age fifty, 50 per cent of all men find themselves in the "occasional difficulties" group, and 10 to 15 per cent are completely unable to achieve a satisfactory erection. These numbers march steadily upwards until age seventy, when over half the male population is unable to stand at attention on demand, or even when not in demand but just hopeful. On the bright side, the Massachusetts Male Aging Study found that 40 per cent of men were still completely potent at age seventy, and yo guys! that's the gang I'm aiming to join.

These numbers are a few years old, by the way, and it's likely that they will be far worse for our male heirs, far too many of whom are too fat, and who will consequently suffer much earlier artery damage and its resultant consequences (see below) than we, their dads, did. This was the main inducement, by the way, for my sons to exercise regularly and keep their weights down. "Vigour, not Viagra" is the new Hister family motto.

In older men, everyone agrees that ED is mostly a physical problem, nearly always caused by damage to the arteries that feed the penis. It's not surprising, then, that erectile difficulties are a lot more common in men who smoke (smokers get ED at much younger ages than nonsmokers, and they tend to get it more severely) and in men who drink heavily. ED is, as everything is, more common in the obese, but happily, one study found that obese men who lose weight can count on regaining their sexual potency.

ED also occurs much more commonly and earlier in men whose arteries are under attack from diseases such as diabetes (ED is extremely common in diabetes), high blood pressure (ditto! one study estimated that at least 70 per cent of men with high blood pressure suffer from ED), and coronary heart disease (a condition that can also produce ED because of a psychological block from a severe fear of dying from any physical exertion, what used to be known as a cardiac cripple). In fact, ED is so prevalent in all these cardiac-connected conditions that any man who begins to suffer increasing bouts of ED must—I repeat, must—consult his doctor about getting checked for diabetes, high blood pressure, and heart disease. This is mandatory because from all the studies that have been done on men who've come forward to ask for ED drugs, we've learned that ED is very often a marker for cardiovascular disease that has not shown up with other symptoms.

Various metabolic, urologic, and neurologic conditions can also lead to ED, and men dealing with chronic health problems are also more prone to ED, both from the psychological burden and from the physical toll that chronic illness exacts. In addition, many medications, especially the kinds of drugs elderly gents need, can affect a man's ability to perform in the only arena that ever matters to most men.

And although I very much believe that exercise is the key to maintaining erectile abilities, I must point out that one other important potential cause of ED is biking. All forms of biking, including mountain biking and long-distance biking, have been associated with an increased risk of ED, probably from the pressure that is exerted on the nerves around the scrotum. Or as my son the economics major put it when I told him to be careful about his future pleasure and my future progeny, " 'Numb nuts equal wilting willie.' Right, Dad?" He's such a bright boy, don't you think?

Finally, that small proportion of men with very low testosterone levels also suffers from ED, although there is still a great deal of debate about the exact relationship between testosterone levels and potency (see below).

In younger men, the situation is quite different because psychological factors, most notoriously fear of failure, play a much larger role in producing ED for that age group than for older men. The Massachusetts Male Aging Study found a link between ED and depression, and perversely, the drugs used to treat depression can also lead to ED, so if you're not suffering with ED when you get depressed, you may start suffering from it as your depression improves, which would be enough to make some men get re-depressed, of course.

Studies have also found a link between ED and repressed anger, as well as between ED and increased stress. For example, Israeli researcher Dr. Alexander Oshanyesky found that when the stock market plummets, so do men's erections, probably because, he told the London *Times*, "stress causes the adrenalin level to shoot up, moving more blood to the brain and the heart and less to the penis," an observation, by the way, that gives the lie to the claim by so many women that a man's heart never has any connection to his penis. See, it clearly does. Also, according to Oshanyesky, there have been only two occasions when an effective drug for ED did not have the desired effect on the men in his Israeli clinic: when Scud missiles hit Israel during the Gulf War, and during the Tel Aviv stock market crash of 1993. But what I really want to know is, what kind of man seeks out this kind of medication when Scud missiles are raining down on his country?

As to treatment, as always, an ounce of prevention is worth a pound of loin, and to that end, I want to make special note of the benefits of exercise in both preventing and treating already established ED. If you exercise enough, several studies have shown that you will have a much lower risk of getting ED in the first place, and if you are already suffering from early ED, then becoming more active has been shown to work as effectively as the drugs that will be discussed below, although it takes the exercise much longer to kick in. And although the exercise may take longer, it also offers you many more benefits, not the least of which is that you don't have to rely on drugs for the rest of your life every time you feel you want to do it.

Otherwise, to prevent ED all the usual lifestyle prohibitions apply. Hard as it may be to follow such guidelines, if you want to minimize softening with age, don't smoke, don't drink too much alcohol (alcohol has a paradoxical effect on sex: it stimulates the brain to want more at the same time that it reduces the body's ability to get what it's seeking), don't become fat, and don't stay sedentary. After all, if you're fat, smoke a ton, drink excessively, and smell like a smoky wino (my wife's nose can spot a smoker at a hundred yards), you will likely get very few chances to find out if you even have an erectile problem in the first place. Also, if you are one of those immature guys who are still using recreational drugs at age fifty, not only do you seriously need a life, man, but until you get one, remember that overuse of all recreational drugs is linked to erectile problems. Bummer, dude.

In addition, be aware that use of some non-recreational drugs also raises the risk of ED. Among the many drugs that can either produce or worsen an already existing softness around the edge, the antihypertensives are especially likely to produce this effect, although digoxin, nonsteroidal anti-inflammatories, antihistamines, tranquillizers, antidepressants, and a host of others can also cause or worsen erectile difficulties, as well as adversely affecting libido. A warning, though: if you suspect that a drug you are on is leaving you limp or lustless in Seattle, don't just stop it abruptly. Talk to your doctor first about perhaps switching to something that might affect you less.

As for most organs, a "use it or lose it" policy is best for the penis too. It's just like riding a bike, you see. Even if you never quite forget how to do it, it's a lot easier to maintain your expertise, especially in traffic, than to go back and do it after a prolonged period of abstinence. Happily, this is the kind of homework most men don't resent doing.

You should also work on stress relief, but remember that ED is not the kind of problem that you can will away. In fact, the more you focus on your inability to perform when Chip is down, the more likely you will be unable to rise the next time out. And remember that in many instances, sexual difficulties, including ED, stem from and are always worsened by communication problems in a relationship, so if you have such problems, consider consulting a professional therapist who is willing to see both you and your patient partner to help you sort things out.

For more active treatment, every culture has witch doctors who promote some sort of aphrodisiac for its underachievers. I don't know what kind of a man would ever resort to trying some of these ridiculous suggestions, but among the many products I have heard about as being effective aphrodisiacs are ginseng, deer antler extract, tiger penises, avocados, rhinoceros horns, carrots, oysters, pomegranates, honey, royal jelly, fertilized duck eggs, lobsters, caviar, prairie oysters or bulls' and rams' testicles (I found those a bit chewy, by the way), bear meat and bear gallbladder (ditto!), wild yams, licorice, and freeze-dried chicken extract (but a warning about that last one: don't forget to remove the packaging before use). And let us never forget the most famous aphrodisiac of all, namely Spanish fly, which is actually made from dry beetles and should really be avoided because it can cause permanent damage to the genitourinary tract.

The drugs sildenafil (Viagra), tadalafil (Cialis), and vardenafil (Levitra) have revolutionized the treatment of ED. These drugs work by blocking an enzyme called PDE5 that allows blood to flow out of the penis. Thus, when a PDE5 inhibitor is taken, the penis engorges and stays filled until it's done its duty or been sent to bed without supper. ED drugs are successful in 70 to 80 per cent of men who suffer from either physically or psychologically based ED, although some men respond better to one drug than another. If, for example, Viagra hasn't worked for you, you have little to lose (except more money) by trying Cialis or Levitra. Viagra and its clones have led to a social revolution that is benefiting a lot of men and their partners. For a start, hardly anyone these days is afraid to talk about what used to be, pre-Viagra, a totally hidden condition (although as my sons will quickly tell you, younger people are sick of being continuously confronted with seniors' prickly problems). More importantly, this new familiarity and ease with ED has led millions of men to come forward and announce that they are not performing up to par and that they could use the help of a pill, although according to the manufacturers, only about 15 per cent of all men who could benefit from ED drugs are getting them. In other words, despite the hoopla and ubiquitous ads with smiling middle-aged (never old) men with nothing better to do than pimp their problem, and despite the ease of therapy (What, after all, could be simpler than swallowing a pill, even for a guy?), 85 per cent of men with ED are not getting treated yet. What, I wonder, is holding those guys back? Shyness? Fear? Or perhaps, dare I suggest, ED is not as big a problem for many men as the pharmaceutical companies would have us believe.

What's the difference among these drugs? Not much. Levitra has the fastest onset of action—something that most men with ED are said to desire greatly: after all, what male ever wants to wait around to shoot after the gun is loaded? So with Levitra, ten to fifteen minutes after a swallow, and you're ready for bear. The others take somewhat longer, up to forty-five minutes for Viagra (although many men respond more quickly), but when you think about it, that's not a real drawback since that's time that could be well spent getting closer to your partner.

The other main difference is that compared to Viagra and Levitra, which work for roughly one night's worth of pleasure (give or take a few hours), Cialis provides what drug company literature likes to call a larger "window of opportunity," but which you and I would call "more time for sex," meaning that it can work for up to thirty-six hours (longer in some men) after ingestion. No wonder, then, that Cialis was quickly labelled "le Weekend" by French men, who have the world's longest weekends anyway. (Ever tried getting anything serviced in France on samedi or dimanche? Actually, ever tried getting anything serviced any other day of the week? "Pas mon job, monsieur.")

Levitra and Cialis can also be taken in more natural circumstances, that is, after ingestion of a full fat meal, while Viagra works fastest if taken on an empty stomach.

Otherwise, there's not that much to choose between them except for a slightly different risk of side effects (see below), so it's really best to pick one that meets your risk profile, try it for as long as you need, and if and when it doesn't work out, then try another one. You can also, of course, always start with a placebo instead of one of these drugs, since in all the studies done on PDE5 inhibitors, placebos also had a very high efficacy rate, as well as a very low rate of side effects. Only thing, your partner shouldn't tell you it's a placebo unless, that is, she wants a quiet night.

Common side effects that have been associated with the use of all these drugs include nuisance problems such as headaches, nausea, abdominal upset, muscular aches and pains, runny nose, dizziness, and diarrhea. Also, as always, be aware that these drugs can interact with other drugs you may be taking, such as alpha blockers, for example, or the antibiotic erythromycin, or HIV medications.

A more serious problem that was reported quite a bit when Viagra first came out was abnormal vision, in which a small proportion of men who take Viagra (this happens with Levitra, too, but not with Cialis), especially those taking higher doses, experience a change in their perception of colour and brightness, and they develop a "bluish" vision. Happily, this seems to be nearly always a transient problem, and has not yet been linked with any adverse long-term effects.

As I write this, however, the U.S. FDA has announced that it has received as many as fifty reports of men who have permanently lost some vision after using PDE5 drugs, mostly Viagra, although that may only be because Viagra has been out there so much longer than the others. The type of vision loss suffered by these men is known as NAION, or non-arteritic anterior ischemic optic neuropathy, and is caused by blood flow to the optic nerve being blocked. So did these men prove your mom right and they went blind suddenly because they were trying to have too much sex? (When I was six or seven, my mom once pointed out a man with shaking hands on the street and said, "See, that's what's going to happen to you." I had no idea what she was talking about but I still remember that guy most days. Actually, most nights.) Or were they simply very sick men to begin with who were at much higher risk of NAION in the first place (both diabetes and heart disease lead to a higher risk of NAION), and the drugs were merely innocent passengers on the train that would have delivered this loss of vision to these guys anyway? It's still far too early to say, although the obvious lesson is that no drug is risk-free, and sometimes we don't learn about serious side effects and complications until a drug has been on the market for many years (say hello to Vioxx, fen-phen, HRT for menopause, and a host of others).

Another serious potential problem is that PDE5 inhibitors lower blood pressure, and although they have been found to be safe in men on high blood pressure drugs, the drop in blood pressure can be precipitous and life-threatening in men who are taking nitroglycerin or other nitrates for angina (chest pain as a result of activity or effort). Thus, men on nitrates must avoid ED drugs. As well, other men who should get a full medical clearance from their doctor before using ED drugs include older men (the older a male, the more hidden heart disease he may have), men with known pre-existing significant heart disease, men with recent heart attacks, men with kidney disease, men with certain eye conditions, and men with low blood pressure.

Another serious albeit rare problem associated with the use of ED drugs and one that's been the butt of many late night comedy skits is priapism, which refers to a penis that, like a bad dog, just won't sit, and gives the owner a prolonged erection lasting at least four hours. Now, I realize that most men reading this will instantly shrug their slight shoulders and mutter, "Well, hey, wouldn't bother me, you know," but you'd be wrong to believe that because priapism is at best an uncomfortable problem (after all, what are you going to do with it after the first bit of fun?) and at worst (thankfully a very rare occurrence) it's a problem that can only be cured with—please sit down before reading on—an operation that destroys the ability to get another erection.

I must also note one other problem associated with ED drugs that is drawing increasing attention, and that is the issue of abuse. In pre-release studies, some men who took Viagra were able to become erect three times a night, which led some experts to worry about the "potential for abuse" or "addiction." Although when I wrote the first edition of *Midlife Man* I argued that this is not really abuse where I come from, I must say that to an extent this concern has proved valid. If some recent surveys are to be believed, Viagra and its clones are indeed being abused by young men, especially gay men, it seems, who don't actually suffer from ED but who are convinced that ED drugs enhance the quality of their erections, the latency period between erections, and hence the satisfaction of their couplings. Even worse, they generally combine these drugs with stimulants and other party drugs, and the result has been a significant rise in unprotected sex and a corresponding rise in sexually transmitted diseases in some parts of the gay community. Clearly, I was wrong: anything that can be used will also one day be abused.

Overall, PDE5 inhibitors are very safe medications that have benefited millions of men and their partners. But if these drugs are safe and effective for the vast majority of men and if, as pointed out earlier, ED is a progressive problem, the question is, why shouldn't all midlifers run out and get some Viagra or Levitra, "just, you know, to get a head start"? Surprisingly, that may just be the advice you do get from your doctor one day, if recent studies pan out. These small and preliminary studies have indicated that ED drugs might have a long-lasting benefit of increased elasticity in all blood vessels, not just the ones you are most concerned about when you get a prescription for one of these drugs.

For now, however, these drugs should still be used only for the treatment of ED, and happily, most of us don't need erectile enhancement—yet—so we have little to gain from using such drugs. Also bear in mind that ED drugs are not like oysters or bulls' testicles: that is, they are not aphrodisiacs and they don't work in the absence of sexual stimulation. For the average midlife guy who's suffering more from sexual boredom than from penile plunging problems, these drugs have little to offer.

Equally important, these drugs do only one thing for their users, to wit: they get the machine primed. But the older I get the more I understand that sexual performance is not the same as sexual intimacy, and that the male obsession with performance to the exclusion of the rest of what is essential for a vital and healthy sexual relationship leads to avoidable trouble in many relationships. The ram in the bedroom may not be as welcome to the ewe as he thinks. In a great column for the *New York Times* that came out when Viagra was first introduced, Maureen Dowd claimed that "what's wrong with these would-be studs [who bought Viagra in the first week it was out] pills can't fix." She went on to say, "An unscientific poll of my girl-friends found that they would rather have a pill that could change a man's personality an hour *after* sex. A pill that insures that he always calls the next day and never gets spooked." Now that ED drugs have been available for several years, I'm sure that most women would probably still agree with that.

A final word of caution from a man who worries about you: if you do decide to use an ED drug, don't get your supply on the Internet because a recent study found that about half the "Viagra" sold on the Internet was not really Viagra, and that many of the pills contained, well, the researchers weren't sure what some of them contained but it certainly wasn't sildenafil.

Also, don't be fooled by those claims about the potential benefits of "herbal Viagras." No such animal, or rather vegetable, exists I'm afraid.

For those who can't or won't take ED drugs, you can, like so many men do, try taking yohimbine, although studies have failed to find it effective (but hey, if it works for you, it works for you because one must never question the placebo effect in improving sexual functioning). Other therapies include phentolamine and zinc. Testosterone replacement therapy may help men with low testosterone levels regain erections (there is still lots of debate about what it does for men with normal testosterone levels), although bear in mind that testosterone replacement also increases the urge to try to barge into areas where you know you should only tread softly.

Of note, nitroglycerin received a standing ovation in at least one report from England in which four of ten men got an erection within two hours of applying a nitro patch, and they were able to maintain their erections for up to three hours. The only significant side effects were headaches and an unfortunate tendency to explode if the subjects wandered too close to an open flame (just kidding about the last).

Pellets of alprostadil that are prodded more than an inch into the urethra are also pushed—gently, I hope—as an effective ED therapy, although studies reveal that in many men this approach doesn't produce the quality of erection required to make the recipient very happy.

And when all else fails, there is still room for some kind of mechanical solution—vacuum suction cylinders, surgically implanted penile inflatable prostheses, and injections.

Finally, a word about something you should not do to try to improve your sexual performance. According to a survey from McGill University reported in the *Medical Post,* "a bigger penis does not cure ED." (It's great to see, by the way, that my alma mater is still on the cutting edge of science.) But what the hell does that mean, you are no doubt wondering. Not what you think. What it means is that cosmetic surgery to enlarge the penis as well as techniques in which the veins to the penis are tied off in an attempt to get blood to stay in the penis longer do not correct erectile difficulties or sexual problems. In fact, if you do have what you consider to be a small penis, take heart in a couple of observations. First, even most smaller penises are still big enough to do whatever jobs they are given. In fact, a recent survey found that although 50 per cent of men desired a bigger penis (to what end, I wonder), nearly 90 per cent of women thought their partner's penis was big enough. Yo, guys, big enough is all that should matter. Second, a recent theory has proposed that body parts may compete for size during development, so the good news is that your smaller penis may simply be a reflection of your larger brain. Or maybe just your larger spleen. Whatever.

Rates of Sexual Intercourse—Liar, Liar

The common belief is that frequency of sexual intercourse slips, generally bit by bit, but occasionally much more dramatically, as we age, a belief that is borne out in most surveys. But before you get too melancholy about a middle and old age restricted to checkers and reruns of *Everybody Loves Raymond,* bear in mind that in surveys about sex there is always an "on the other hand." So on the other hand, I have seen at least three encouraging surveys. One found that 30 per cent of men over the age of eighty claimed they were still having intercourse at least once a week (my son said he didn't really want to think about that). A second survey for the American Association for Retired Persons found that 51 per cent of all respondents claimed to be "extremely" or "somewhat" happy with their sex lives, which doesn't tell you much about frequency but does tell you that sexual satisfaction doesn't really have to drop that much with age, and that's really what it's all about, isn't it. Of course, old, retired people may be more easily pleased than younger people are, but I don't want to think about that. And the third study found that one Canadian man in five over the age of seventy says he's still having sex weekly. That's weekly, and not weakly, by the way, although it's often both, of course.

I must warn you to take this latter survey with a grain of salt, though, because it also found that only one Canadian woman in fifteen over age seventy said that she was having sex weekly. So how can we explain this discrepancy between the Canuck old guys and gals? The possibilities are 1) that one in five elderly Canadian men is a liar (impossible!), 2) that those geezers are bedding younger women in droves (also hard to believe considering what our hordes of grizzled, pucklike, tuque-wearing, older gents look like), 3) that they are having sex with each other (perish the thought), or 4) that they are having lots of virtual sex or, most likely, lots of sex with themselves, which makes me wonder in turn about the 80 per cent of Canadian senior men who aren't even up to doing that.

But no matter what the numbers say, the important point is that sex surveys have very little relevance for thee and me because how frequently each of us has sexual intercourse depends on many factors (some of which we can control, some of which we can't) that affect each of us differently. For a start, for most of us, sexual intercourse tends to occur much more often if we have a partner. As we men age, however, our ability to hang on to a partner, or to discover a new partner, willing to do it as often as we want to do it, is more difficult than it was when we were younger.

Men who are depressed or under lots of stress or who suffer from other psychological problems also tend to have (and tend to want to have) much less intercourse than their carefree, play-it-as-it-lays brothers. Other factors that have been shown to affect the frequency at which all men, not just the middle-aged, have sexual intercourse are:

- employment status: clearly, having a job helps you get a partner
- income level: generally the more money you have in the bank, the more sex you can bank on
- neurological and brain changes that occur inevitably with advancing age: these changes include alterations in the levels of some neurotransmitters in the brain
- education level: a recent survey found that contrary to what you may think, the more education you achieve, the less sex you have, a finding that nearly convinced one of my sons to quit school until I told him he could get the same results by pretending to any new girls he meets that he never finished high school (something he can fake rather easily, unfortunately)
- what we own: gun owners, jazz CD owners, and trailer owners report having more sex than we peace-loving, nonhip homeowners do, thus answering the age-old poser of why anyone would ever buy a trailer
- the state of our health and the state of our partners' health: frequency of intercourse generally declines in direct proportion to the illnesses we develop
- the worries we have about our health: some guys are simply petrified of anything that might increase their heart rate the least bit, and for most guys, sexual intercourse leads to a spike in heart rate, for a few seconds anyway

So take heart in knowing that for the individual, statistics about the frequency of sexual intercourse mean absolutely nothing. There are too many variables to know what your future will bring. That said, if you're a jazz-loving, gun-toting, uneducated trailer park resident, there's a very good chance you will be boinking your way frequently and happily into old age. Then again, maybe not. But hey, don't worry about it because that will only make the problem worse.

Sex, Chickens, Golf, and Death—the Four Horsemen of the Jewish Apocalypse

Statistics and surveys aside, common sense tells me that for the great majority of men, the frequency of sexual intercourse is likely to decrease significantly with age. Why? For a start, most men tend to become monogamous with age, usually willingly, occasionally not, and although monogamy has much to recommend it—it is certainly easier on the nerves, for example—monogamy also breeds a sexual constancy, a certain stuck-in-the-same-way mind set and body set that can easily allow a couple's sexual relationship to be taken for granted and consequently become increasingly ignored or passed over in favour of other pleasures or activities.

In that way, the history of the average couple's sex life is similar to the history of my passion for roast chicken. When I was young and had just flown my mother's coop, nothing used to fire up my taste buds as much as the smell of a newly roasted kosher capon cooking in the oven. But now that I'm older, a roasting, sweet-smelling bird no longer stimulates my salivary glands the way it once did. I do still eat lots of roast chicken, of course, especially when it's dressed in a new and beguiling manner, but not as often as I once did. And while there's nothing like a new spice on an old hen to whet the flagging appetite, nature, I have been told, has not yet come up with a comparable ruse to fool a hen into thinking an old rooster is just as desirable as he used to be.

And so it is with sex. Thus I'm not surprised that according to a Japanese survey, one in three Japanese couples doesn't have sex, while a British survey found that one in ten seemingly happy couples between the ages of forty-five and fifty-nine abstain from sexual relations, not for religious reasons, but through an agreement that there is simply something better to do with their time. What they didn't say is what that something better is, but hey, it may be worth trying to find out.

There's more at work in aging men, however, than just constancy on the home front to temper their urge to have sexual intercourse as frequently as they claim they had it when they were younger. For example, when an aging man turns away from the pursuit of intercourse as his only goal in a sexual relationship, he is often able to work on developing a stronger nonsexual intimacy and bond with his partner. This improvement in his marriage increases his chances of having crucial social support later in life when he will really need it.

Also, as men get older, we need to take more time and energy to get everything working in the right order, and we are forced to invest more time and effort in doing many things that used to come much more easily. Sex is no exception. Since we have only so much energy to spare, many conclude, consciously or not, that they would rather invest their limited capacities in something that is much easier to manage than sex and that, on the whole, is more likely to offer a positive psychological return for their effort. That's why, of course, so many middle-aged men have taken up golf, which after all, is merely the modern-day equivalent of male bonding through hunting—you golf with your buddies, women are usually excluded, you (occasionally) bring back a trophy your wife has no idea what to do with, you golf outdoors, you use clubs, you dress like an idiot, and so on. And golf is also easier on the psyche and the ego than sex is. After all, your golfing abilities don't tail off as you hit your middle years; no one laughs at you if you are the one with the shortest putts; if the earth moves while you're making a golf shot, you don't have to wait forever to try it again but rather, you get to do it over right away; and most important, when you golf you can really relax because you never have to worry if your partners are enjoying it as much as you are. So for many middle-aged guys, the pursuit of birdies has replaced the pursuit of birds.

But there's also this: a drop-off in sex as men age may be what nature intended. "Huh?" I can hear a few of you guys saying over that beer you've just spilled. "Why would nature be so cruel?" Because less frequent sex may help men live longer and better. You see, evolutionists tell us that there are only so many resources and just so much energy an organism has to spend on its four vital needs: growth, maintenance and repair, storage, and reproduction, so the more an organism spends in one area, the less it has to spend in other areas. It should be no surprise, then, that studies have linked a higher rate of sexual activity in males of many species to earlier death. For example, a study on male marsupial mice who spend—I hope you're sitting down for this, guys—from five to eleven hours a day copulating (foreplay is very, very short, though, and pretty impersonal) found that castrated marsupial male mice live much longer, on average, than the uncastrated ones.

British scientist David Gems from London's University College reviewed animal studies on sex and longevity and concluded, the *New Scientist* reports, that males of many species would outlive females if only the males could temper their sex drive. As a specific example, male nematode worms that were separated from females increased their life spans from ten days to twenty days, double the life expectancy for the average male, as well as four days longer than the average life expectancy of female nematode worms. So the next time your mate rolls over and says, "Not tonight, dear, I want you to live longer," better believe that she's only doing it for your own good. At least that's what my wife tells me, but I think it's probably more because she wants to live longer.

The key question, though, is this: what killer effect might sexual activity exert on a male nematode worm? The most popular theory is that non-sex-seeking worms don't actually live longer, they just feel as if they've lived longer. The more scientific theory is that males that don't seek sex may live longer because they tend to move around less than their sex-seeking brothers—that is, the shy guys don't waste a lot of energy competing with other males or defending worm territory, a theory that won't surprise anyone who has ever watched human male worms competing with each other in a singles bar. Talk about a waste of energy.

More weight to the less sex–longer life theory comes from researchers at the California Institute of Technology, who recently concluded that primate males such as the mountain gorilla, who share at least some of the parenting duties, seem to live nearly as long as the females. In contrast, primate males such as the chimpanzee, who play little or no role in parenting the young, tend to die significantly earlier than the females of that species. What does that have to do with sex? you are no doubt wondering. It seems to me that human males are much more like gorillas than chimpanzees (lots of women would say "for sure" to that), so it may pay men—they will live longer for it—to stay in family units and care for their young. The cost, as I already said, is probably less frequent, home-based sex, but the benefit is a longer and, I submit, happier life.

Thus, it may be that less frequent pursuit of sex as we age is just healthier in the long run, although it's always wise to remember that as John Maynard Keynes said, "in the long run, we are all dead."

Premature Ejaculation—Too Ready for Prime Time

As I sat down to write this, I couldn't help but remember the unique voice of my high school gym teacher, who always used to lament the fact that he was stuck with me in his classes, and who would often shrug and mutter, "PE is just not for you, Hister." And happily, he was right, but not how he meant it.

Premature ejaculation, or PE, is one of those problems that is much in the eyes of the beholder (or the one being beheld) because clearly the speed at which a man delivers his load matters only to him and his partner, so whereas some men and their partners are happy with a Domino's pizza relationship, that is, a very speedy delivery (or the next time it's free?), others are unhappy with even a very slow amble to the summit.

That said, doctors need to quantify everything in order to treat it, so to that end a recent study (sponsored by a company that's dying to bring out a pill to treat PE, please note) determined that the average time from start to finish for men is about seven minutes (for women, it's about a week), but when it comes to satisfying most men and their partners, two minutes—from entry to deposit—is the minimum amount of time needed.

Thus, it is soon bound to become customary, I am sure, to declare that anything under two minutes constitutes PE (although clearly, some men and their partners won't be happy unless the man is able to delay deposit and detumescence until the proverbial cows come home, and not even then, for some), and with this definition, PE turns out to be a very common condition, with 30 to 35 per cent of men coming in under that magical two minutes. Interestingly, in cultures where speed in delivery is thought to be a measure of manhood (think the Middle East, of course), this definition of PE is greeted with a great deal of derision.

The good news for the too-fast-for-thee boys who live in North America and not Iraq is that there will soon be drugs available to help them slow down. This has all come about from the observation that some men on SSRI antidepressants such as fluoxetine (Prozac) and sertraline (Zoloft) experience a slowing in their time to climax. Of course, a lot of men put on these drugs experience a total cessation of climax since the drugs often lower libido, too, but that's another matter. Building on that information, researchers have developed a pill in the SSRI family called dapoxetine that is in later trials now for the treatment of PE. And how effective is it?

According to the trial that came out just as this book went to press, men who started with what the experts call an intravaginal ejaculatory latency time (you and I would say it's the time it takes a man to come) of forty-five to fifty-five seconds were able to extend that to 2.3 minutes, on average, and although that may not sound like such a huge extension to some of you, most men in this study and their partners claimed a significantly higher rate of sexual satisfaction after taking the pills.

There may still be a rub to this one, though, because 10 per cent of men in this study suffered significant side effects from dapoxetine, including such symptoms as nausea, headache, diarrhea, and dizziness.

It's also important to note that the men on placebo in this trial went from fifty seconds on average to nearly two minutes, so as with most matters to do with male sexual functioning, a major part of the problem in PE is clearly in the mind. Fool them and they will come.

Testosterone—Why Men Will Always Be Boys

Testosterone is the hormone that deepens a young boy's voice, puts hair on his chest and face, and gives him his manly physique—more manly, of course, in some cases (e.g., Mike Tyson) than in others (e.g., Richard Simmons). In short, testosterone is what turns a male into a real man. Although it is often referred to as "the male sex hormone," all of us—men, women, and the in-between—secrete some testosterone; men just secrete more of it.

Testosterone starts its work early in fetal life, when it is responsible for the development of the male genitalia and male reproductive organs, and when it is also responsible for starting the masculinization of the male brain, which is what determines that a boy will want a gun in his hands as soon as he can stand and that he will eventually feel a constant need to bang some two-by-fours together to build a deck while drinking beer.

After birth, testosterone lies low until puberty, when a sudden huge hormone hurricane not only leads to maturation and growth of the male reproductive apparatus but also produces a change that we all dread when it rears its untamable head in adolescent boys: their sudden and intense interest in S E X. And I do mean intense. If you've ever owned one, you undoubtedly have learned that the typical adolescent boy is often nothing more than an out-of-control hormone-hijacked vehicle, and he gets little relief from his hormones even during sleep, when his wet dreams often become the cause of next-morning embarrassment for both him and his parents.

Testosterone production also rises significantly in adolescent girls, although clearly not nearly to the same extent as it pours into pubescent boys' circulation. Why are adolescent girls also subjected to a testosterone gusher? Because testosterone is essential to kick off two well-known and corresponding evolutionarily driven phenomena: the teenage girl's sex drive, and her father's urge to buy himself a shotgun.

Testosterone Factories—Location and Function

Most testosterone is produced in the testicles, where special cells manufacture the hormone from cholesterol. A small amount of testosterone is also produced in the adrenal glands, which make it in much the same manner as the testicles do. Testosterone-producing cells either make their own cholesterol or grab some of the circulating cholesterol that's all around them, so you clearly need a lot of the cholesterol that you have circulating in you; without it, you will end up spending too much time watching the Shopping Channel. And cholesterol is something most men need to feel easy about because these days it is usually portrayed as the guy in the black hat come to drive the life out of Dodge by plugging all the arteries in town with fat. But cholesterol also plays a very important role in many essential functions, some of which may be adversely affected when a man lowers his cholesterol count precipitously. For example, if a man allows his wife to pester him into going on a low-fat diet (the only reason most middle-aged men will ever go on a low-fat diet) and as a result his cholesterol count drops significantly, he may, according to at least one study, also suffer a corresponding drop in his testosterone production, which would, of course, allow his wife to boss him around even more.

All the steps in testosterone synthesis are under the control of the hypothalamus, the *überstampführer* of the endocrine system. The hypothalamus discharges its duty by constantly monitoring signals from body tissues and organs that tell it how much testosterone is required for current needs. For example, if a man is getting ready to go bear hunting or in-law visiting, equivalently stressful events for most guys, he clearly needs a quick preemptive hit of testosterone to help him make it through such a stressful event. In anticipation, the hypothalamus secretes a chemical called gonadotropin-releasing hormone (GRH), which heads straight to the pituitary gland and primes it to secrete luteinizing hormone (LH) and follicle-stimulating hormone (FSH). LH stimulates the testicles to produce testosterone, while FSH initiates the production of sperm—although the sperm are clearly not as necessary on a bear shoot or a visit to the in-laws as is the extra testosterone. At least I hope not.

Testosterone Levels—One Man's Ceiling Is Another Man's Floor

Normal levels of circulating testosterone range from 10.4 to 41.6 nmol/L (300 to 1,200 ng/dL). You would immediately assume, then, that a man with a testosterone level of 40.0 nmol/L is twice as likely to want to go to war as a guy with a reading of 20.0 nmol/L. Wrong, wrong, wrong. In fact, most doctors consider the two men to be equal in all essential measures of manliness with equal levels of aversion to in-laws, equal reluctance to consult a map even when hopelessly lost, and equal need to belch and slap butt. Why? Well, since nearly all circulating testosterone travelling in the blood is bound to carrier proteins, including albumin and sex-hormone-binding globulin (SHBG), circulating testosterone is relatively inactive and unavailable to the tissues (think of testosterone as one of those smallish cars that you so often see tied to the back of some oversized, cigar-shaped, highway-hogging, lawnchair-toting RV that always seems to be in front of you on a one-lane highway). As a result, large variations in circulating testosterone levels actually translate into little difference in "maleness"—that is, in testosterone's effects on the tissues and organs and brain.

There's something else that's also very important to know about testosterone tests, which explains that wide range of normal values—namely, that levels can fluctuate dramatically in an individual man, both in the short term and in the long term, depending on many variables. Unlike your commitment to your team, to your dog, or even to your true love, your testosterone level is not constant and unchanging even on a given day, and depending on when it's taken and what you are up to, the reading may vary significantly. Thus, for example, testosterone levels tend to be higher in single men and drop when these men hitch up. A man's testosterone level may also fall when he is laid off work and, as already noted, when he eats a low-fat diet. Testosterone level is also affected by the seasons—it tends to be highest in the fall and lowest in the spring when a man's fancy turns to, well, it never really turns, does it?—and even by the time of day (it falls during the day, rises at night—*quelle surprise*—and is highest early in the morning). Your mood and your personality also play a role. Thus, as you would expect, trial lawyers have higher testosterone levels than their non-litigating colleagues. It has also been shown that a man's testosterone level tends to shoot upwards when his team wins an important match and it goes down when his team loses, which explains a lot about me, I'm afraid, since the team I root for, the Chicago Cubs, hasn't won a World Series since Theodore Roosevelt was president of the United States.

Now, clearly, most of the aforementioned factors generally lead to only small fluctuations in testosterone levels, but they can add up, so all that has to be taken into account when getting a one-off testosterone test. And then there's the crucial effect of age. Starting at around age forty, a man's testosterone level tends to drop slowly but gradually, in part because of rising levels of sex-hormone-binding globulin, which begins to sop up increasing amounts of testosterone.

How fast and how much testosterone declines, however, varies significantly from man to man for reasons that are still not clear. One variable may be personality. Thus, according to a study from the University of Pittsburgh, Type A men, who are described as driven, aggressive, and combative (Hell, I'm not combative!), show a greater decline in testosterone levels with age than do their Type B "let-me-stop-to-smell-the-flowers-and-while-I'm-at-it-let-me-also-take-a-nap-in-the-flower-bed-cuz-it's-just-such-a-doo-da-great-world" brothers.

Lifestyle factors may also play a role. This same study also found that the more a man smokes over a lifetime and the lower his dietary fat intake, the more his testosterone level tends to fall with age. Also, a recent study has linked Type II diabetes with significantly lower testosterone levels, and since Type II diabetes is largely a disorder of too much weight and too little exercise, it stands to reason that doing more exercise and controlling weight might also keep testosterone levels up.

Because of the difficulty in interpreting testosterone levels, many researchers now believe that a more accurate gauge of testosterone's real effects is the level of "free" testosterone, which is testosterone that is not bound to a carrier protein and which is thus much more available to the tissues. Free testosterone makes up about 2 per cent of all the circulating testosterone.

So what happens to free testosterone with age? It, too, drops significantly as we get older. According to research by Dr. John Morley, half of all men between the ages of fifty and seventy have free testosterone levels below the lowest level seen in healthy men between the ages of twenty and forty.

The preceding observation about falling levels of testosterone and free testosterone with age leads us to some very big questions that will concern every man reading this book:

- Is this drop in testosterone and free testosterone with age an unnatural process that should be averted with any means at our disposal?
- Or is this drop in hormones simply nature's way of telling you that you're not a young man anymore and you shouldn't really try to be?
- Even if we establish that it's better to have higher testosterone levels, do we really know how to boost those levels?
- And even if we can boost testosterone levels effectively, how do we know that the testosterone is hitting the target organs it's intended to hit or that it's even safe?

And you thought this would be an easy Sunday-drive read, eh?

Why Arnold Schwarzenegger Has a Female Side Too

When it hits the tissues, testosterone must first get converted to other hormones, such as 5-alpha-dihydrotestosterone, which do the actual masculinizing work on the tissues. It may come as a surprise to learn that one of the hormones to which testosterone is converted—I don't know how to break this gently, guys—is estrogen, a conversion that would make even my rabbi proud. What it means is that Arnold Schwarzenegger, Russell Crowe, Dick "Mine are bigger than yours" Cheney, even Don Cherry—every man, whether he chooses to recognize his feminine side or whether he is so scared of it that he is at all times determined to impress us with his over-the-top masculinity—has at least some estrogen circulating in his bloodstream. And this estrogen is very important because this "female" hormone apparently helps sperm to mature. "So what else is new—don't men always need help with getting some maturity?" asked a female friend of mine when I told her this bit. You see why women never win Nobel Prizes in science?

Also, and this is not going to shock anyone who's ever seen a seventy-year-old man's breasts jiggle as he takes his shirt off, the rate of conversion of testosterone to estrogen goes up with age, with the amount of fat tissue you have managed to store because fat cells produce estrogen, and with any process (such as excessive alcohol intake and the use of some medications) that damages liver cells and hinders the breakdown of testosterone.

Why Hunters Are Hairy, Lonely, and Bald

Testosterone is a very busy hormone. For example, testosterone is essential for:

- the production of sebum
- the development and maturation of muscles
- hair growth in certain areas, such as the armpits, face, and lower pubis
- bone health: low testosterone levels are linked to a higher risk of osteoporosis
- the production of red blood cells
- nitrogen balance
- calcium balance
- carbohydrate metabolism
- electrolyte balance
- psychological well-being

Testosterone has also been shown to inhibit inflammation, nourish cartilage, and affect visuospatial skills and perceptual abilities. An interesting study in rats has suggested that testosterone might be more effective in preventing Alzheimer's disease than estrogen, thus raising the very scary prospect of all postmenopausal women being urged to take testosterone to protect their brains. Some of us are just not ready for that.

By the way, one of the best ways to illustrate some of the aforementioned effects is to note that when someone is subject to too much testosterone (these effects are generally much more pronounced in women), they develop increased facial hair, oily skin, deepening of the voice, acne, and male-pattern baldness, as well as depression and irritability—but then what woman would not become depressed and irritable if she suddenly became bald, sprouted a bunch of zits, grew a beard, and started singing bass in the church choir?

In the reproduction arena, testosterone's best-known responsibility is to act as the foreman in the assembly-line production of sperm, a major responsibility to be sure, since the average male is said to produce over 100 million sperm a day, an enormous waste of effort given that nearly every one of those little guys is destined to die a quick death either at home or on some foreign battlefield, underemployed and unlamented.

Testosterone is also responsible for male sexual development, especially the growth of the penis at puberty, as well as for the emergence of secondary male sexual characteristics, such as hair growth, deepening of the voice, and pelvis development. In fact, without testosterone, we would all be female, which, despite what the Henry Higginses of the world might tell you, would, in my opinion, not be such a bad thing. The major advantage would be that the world would be much less likely to suffer wars or put up with wife-beating sports stars who nevertheless still earn multi-millions of dollars. The downside, however, would be a world in which there would be nearly constant disputes over the splitting of restaurant bills as well as a world where no kitchen or bathroom was safe from renovation. (I ask you: has any man anywhere ever walked into his home and declared, "Honey, I think the bathroom needs redoing because those fixtures are too old-fashioned"?)

As has already been noted, testosterone also masculinizes brain tissue, starting very early in fetal development. Thus, with the exception of only a few die-hard nonbelievers, we all now realize that there is a great deal of difference between a male infant and a female infant and that much of that difference stems from genetic factors that are simply beyond the parents', or even society's and advertising's, control.

Perhaps the clearest evidence of this difference can be seen if you offer a young boy a doll to play with. Although a few boys will undoubtedly do what nearly all young girls do with the doll, that is, construct some fairy-tale world in which the doll plays a central, and usually a very romantic, role, the typical young boy—even if he has been brought up without television and in a family fervently committed to spiritualism, pacifism (unless you attack our family), and saving of endangered species—will inevitably point the doll at the nearest bystander and yell, "Bang, bang, you're dead." Quieter boys may instead sit there and tear the head off the doll to see what's inside, but then they will point it and yell, "Bang, bang, you're dead."

Social factors undoubtedly play an important role in the development of these different behaviour patterns, but much of the difference between boys and girls is also attributable to the effect of gender-specific hormones on these youngsters' brains and emotions. The problem is that we still don't know much about how these sex hormones affect us, and much of what we thought we knew may not be accurate. It has traditionally been held, for example, that testosterone leads men to be much more aggressive and violent. Thus, when injected with testosterone, lab animals tend to become more aggressive towards their cell mates as well as towards their handlers, trying to bite the fingers off the injector's hand, for example (that is, when they are not busy trying to mount the hand). In addition, prisoners incarcerated for violent crimes have been shown to have higher testosterone levels than the general population. Even female prisoners with higher testosterone levels tend to exhibit more aggressive behaviour in prison than do their convict sisters with lower levels of testosterone, and this aggressive behaviour tends to decrease as their testosterone levels fall with age. But more recent research has indicated that testosterone may be getting a bit of a bad rap, and that aggression and its ugly sibling, violence, may be linked more to estrogen receptors in the brain. In other words, it may be only when testosterone is converted to estrogen that it produces an increased tendency to become aggressive and violent. The political implications of these findings are too much for this man to contemplate.

Testosterone's effects on the cardiovascular system are subject to a great deal of debate. For many years, it had generally been held that since men suffered way more heart attacks and strokes than women and at younger ages, testosterone must somehow be responsible for that raised risk, most likely through a deleterious effect on the levels of blood lipids such as HDL (high-density lipoprotein—the "good" cholesterol) and LDL (low-density lipoprotein—the "bad" cholesterol).

Most experts now argue, however, that this testosterone–heart attack link is a spurious cause-and-effect connection on a par with the claim that drinking milk leads to a higher risk of drug use since nearly all drug addicts drank milk in huge amounts when they were younger. Why the reassessment? First, and most important, we now know that postmenopausal women eventually have just as high a rate of heart disease and strokes as do men. Second, if high testosterone levels really caused an increased number of heart attacks, then the rate of heart attacks in men should drop significantly as men get older and their testosterone levels drop, which is the opposite of what happens. In fact, many experts now believe that a low testosterone level might predispose a man to a higher risk of heart attack, and they advise aging men to take testosterone replacement to lower their risk of heart attack. As evidence for this view, they can cite a recent study that found that teenage boys who had severe acne (presumably because of higher testosterone levels) were significantly less likely to die of heart disease over the following thirty years compared with their zit-free brothers.

So which is it? No one is sure, but the wavering consensus these days seems to be that treatment with testosterone, whether by injection or some other method, has either a neutral or a small beneficial effect on heart attack risk. This is clearly something that needs a lot more study.

Testosterone also has a huge effect on mood and temperament. A study from Iowa, for example, found that men with low testosterone levels had an incidence of mood and anxiety disorders that was three times as high as that of men with normal levels. And a study from the University of California on men with low testosterone levels, who had described themselves as edgy, irritable, and angry, found that after several months those men who were given testosterone injections now described themselves as less angry and agitated as well as happier and more optimistic (although I suspect that a good part of the reason these men were so much happier after the therapy was that they were also having more sex than they had before the injections).

So a low testosterone level does not make for a happy man. But then, curiously, nor does a high testosterone level. The Massachusetts Male Aging Study, for example, found that men with higher levels of testosterone are unhappier and lonelier than men who have lower levels. Why? Because compared with men who have normal or low testosterone levels, high-testosterone men have been found to be more dominant, aggressive, competitive, assertive, "highly interested" in sports (as if this were a bad thing), distant and unsympathetic, and likely to throw temper tantrums.

They are also less likely to get married (no kidding!) and more likely to get divorced if they do hitch up. It should be no surprise, then, that high-testosterone men are also reported to receive less emotional support from family and friends than do their less aggressive brothers. Well, would you want to console that kind of man when he's down? How would you even get close enough to him to know when he's down? Hint: do not try to console him when he's watching his team on the tube, especially when the team's losing.

Testosterone and Sexual Functioning—Priming the Pump

Which finally brings us to the issue that has probably kept most of you reading this far: what about testosterone and sex? How does testosterone, either the endogenous kind, which we make on our own, or the exogenous kind, which is injected or ingested or patched on, affect sex drive, sexual abilities, and the perennial bottom line—frequency of intercourse? The answer is not nearly as simple as you might imagine, because sexual functioning in men is much more complicated than it might seem.

Now I know that to most women, nearly every man seems a hopelessly simple sexual being, an automatonic unrebellious slave to an overexercised imagination and an overprimed, ever-ready, perpetual-motion single-purpose pump—driven upwards and ever more upwards by excessive gobs of testosterone. And I am sure that some men are actually like that. Most men, however, are not. In most guys, testosterone is only one part of what makes us tick sexually. To quote noted hormone researcher Dr. John Morley, "Sexual activity in men is composed of both libido and potency. Libido consists of sexual desire and drive, thoughts, fantasies, satisfaction and pleasure. Potency consists of the ability to obtain and maintain an erection and to ejaculate. Although potency and libido are interdependent, in men sex hormones appear to be predominantly involved in the production of libido." In other words, although testosterone does play a role in the ability to get the apparatus up and working, it plays a much more important role in producing the urge to put that apparatus into play in the first place, which is why testosterone is probably the reason that men think about sex so much more often than women do. And boy, do they ever think about it. A recent survey, for example, found that while women think about sex roughly once a day on average (generally, I guess, while chopping onions), men think of sex about four times a day on average, information that prompted my son to ask, "What do those guys think about the rest of the time?" "About earning a living," I told him, but he was gone before I got the words out.

A man with a very low testosterone level has little sexual desire and is not easily aroused by appropriate sexual stimuli, which for a normal guy is usually simply the smell or sight of a nearby person of the sex he desires, or even a facsimile of same. A man with a very low testosterone level also:

- has fewer erections
- gets hard less often
- stays hard for a shorter period of time
- has fewer nighttime erections (which are an excellent measure, by the way, of whether a man can even get an erection)
- has a smaller volume of ejaculate
- ejaculates less forcefully than men with higher testosterone levels

It's important to note, though, that even men with very low testosterone levels can still get aroused by sufficiently strong sexual stimuli, such as the smell of a new Porsche, and can perform up to par, although I suppose the number of strokes in par is often a matter of dispute.

To summarize testosterone's role in sexual desire and drive, one can say that when testosterone levels are low, men don't think about sex as often; even if they think about it, they don't feel like it; and even if they feel like it, they often can't do it as well. But in the end, they can often still deliver the necessary goods.

Testosterone Replacement Therapy—More Bang for the Buck?

As anyone with an interest in these matters can attest, increasing numbers of experts are popping up in the media urging all middle-aged and older men to get their testosterone levels measured, and if the level is at all "low," to start taking testosterone replacement therapy (TRT). After all, these experts ask, if it does nothing else, wouldn't this exogenous testosterone improve every man's sexual functioning? As always, though, it's not that simple or straightforward.

On the plus side, we know that many men with abnormally low testosterone levels respond well to testosterone replacement therapy. In fact, they very much need it because it lowers their risk of conditions such as osteoporosis and muscle loss, it brings them more energy and better moods, and most important for many of them, it improves their sexual functioning significantly, too. In fact, it's precisely those guys with abnormally low testosterone levels who clearly benefited from testosterone therapy that make up a disproportionately high percentage of all the happy hangers trotted forth in uncontrolled studies and anecdotal reports that tout the benefits of TRT.

But middle-aged men with documented, conclusive, abnormally low testosterone levels make up only a very small percentage of all middle-aged men. What about the much more substantial number of men whose testosterone levels are normal, or even that oxymoronic "low normal," and who have some or all of the symptoms that some experts typically ascribe to andropause (see Chapter 1) or partial androgen deficiency in the aging male (PADAM):

- mood swings
- fatigue
- poorer memory
- difficulty concentrating and decline in other cognitive functions
- increased anxiety
- physical aches and pains
- diminished libido and erectile quality
- decrease in lean body mass (fat replaces muscle)
- decreased strength
- decreased body hair

Is this collection of complaints (in whole or in part) a unique syndrome or do these symptoms merely represent a shopping list of aging? Depends on whom you ask. Thus, the experts who believe in PADAM insist that in the aging male it's very important to recognize PADAM as a distinct entity and to treat it because PADAM is associated with an increased risk of osteoporosis, muscle loss, and perhaps even heart disease and Alzheimer's disease, and that TRT can not only counteract these increased risks but it can also improve most of the symptoms of PADAM, increase muscle strength, improve bone density, and lead to better fat distribution, not to mention the benefits it would bestow on a man's flagging libido and drooping sexual functioning.

Recently, going one step further, an offshoot of this school has lobbied to lower the focus on testosterone replacement and raise the profile of other hormones that should also be added to an aging male's therapy regimen. Thus, for these folks, it's no longer TRT they're pushing on aging men but rather androgen replacement therapy or ART (an acronym I very much like, by the way), which includes any or all of DHEA, growth hormone, melatonin, thyroxin, leptin, and several other hormones that have yet to be discovered in addition to testosterone.

I just don't buy it. Yet.

First, I believe that the symptoms of PADAM are far too vague to constitute a unique syndrome, unless you consider normal aging to be a syndrome, and that the symptoms ascribed to PADAM are really just the ordinary kinds of things we all experience as we age and which have little to do with falling testosterone levels.

But even if we could establish that falling hormone levels contributed somewhat to such symptoms, and that's a very big if, what bothers me most about the PADAM-and-treat school is that we still don't know that trying to prop up declining hormone levels is either beneficial or safe. Perhaps God or Darwin wanted older folks to end up with gradually lower hormone levels for their own protection. It's possible, perhaps even probable, that a lower though still normal testosterone level and its corresponding decrease in sexual drive might just help you live longer and healthier, an evolutionary (or God-mandated) manipulation that forces an often unwilling aging man to stop fighting younger bucks for territory and younger, fertile mates, to whom he really has no attachment. An excessive sexual drive, in other words, might be harmful for an older male. One study from the UK, for example, concluded that having sex with someone who is not your spouse significantly increases the risk of suffering a heart attack and, even worse, the risk of sudden death during sex (yikes!). And older men are, of course, much more prone to heart attacks. Thankfully, most affairs don't end with the male in the coronary care unit but hey, if it does, you're gonna have a lot of "splaining" to do, Lucy. For added proof for this link, we can look at the animal kingdom, specifically, the male junco bird. You see, the higher a male junco's testosterone levels, the more likely this normally monogamous bird is to covet a junco female he has not known before, which clearly leads him into some pretty dangerous territory, and as with junco science, so perhaps with science in humans, too.

Also, men with lower testosterone levels report getting more emotional support from friends and family than do their more aggressive brothers, so perhaps as we get older lower testosterone levels increase our chances of maintaining better social relationships and social support systems, which are known to decrease the risk of premature death. In other words, maybe a lower testosterone level is God's way of keeping a man at home, where he can concentrate on improving his familial relationships and protecting his DNA-bearing offspring (although to be fair, a man can never really tell, can he, which one of those heavy eaters on his couch bears his DNA and which one is an accidental tourist, and besides, most of those heavy eaters do not want or need to be protected).

There's also this that nags at me: because of the feedback loop that testosterone is part of, any outside source of testosterone is likely to affect other hormone levels as well. So what are those other hormones doing when you take TRT? And how does that matter? In one study, middle-aged men who took testosterone all experienced a drop in follicle-stimulating hormone, luteinizing hormone, and sex-hormone-binding globulin. Researchers simply don't know yet what such changes may mean.

Another crucial reason for going slow on testosterone replacement therapy is the still very unanswered question of how it will affect your prostate. Although most studies have indicated that testosterone therapy does not raise the risk of either prostate enlargement or prostate cancer, other studies have linked higher testosterone levels to both prostate enlargement and prostate cancer. Clearly, much better research is needed to tell us exactly what effect TRT has on a man's most intimate gland.

Finally, even if hormones help a bit with some PADAM symptoms, what bothers me is the focus on TRT as the way to deal with them. The key to better health in old age, including the need to keep falling hormone levels as high as possible, should not be hormone replacement but rather a much stronger emphasis on weight control, diet, and exercise. In fact, studies show that you can raise your testosterone levels through natural means. For example, according to an article in *Men's Health*, studies have found higher testosterone levels in weight lifters, serious competitors, and meat eaters versus vegetarians. We also know that testosterone levels tend to drop in men who overexercise and those who sleep fewer hours. My wife, by the way, lifts weights, often sleeps in, and you would never want to face her over a gin rummy hand (although lucky for me, she has recently become a vegetarian).

I know, however, that despite my many objections to this wholesale open-ended experiment on millions of men, that in this hormone-happy world, many men reading this far will still seek some ART, and I can't really blame you, if you do, because we would all like to stay virile and potent and full of ourselves as we were when we were younger. So if you do go after ART (I feel very funny when I put it like that, for some reason, so I'm going to go back to calling it TRT), you should familiarize yourself with all the touted benefits and risks of testosterone and the available methods of getting it: injections, pills, sprays, and patches (no suppository—yet).

So what about those benefits? What can testosterone replacement therapy do for you? At the very least, it will increase your sexual desire because it does that for everyone, even for postmenopausal women who are given testosterone. On the risks side, however, these women also report sudden surges of interest in running out to buy a set of Craftsman tools, but hey, at least those tools last a lifetime. Or so my handymen tell me. As a typical Jewish man, you see, I have no tools—only a set of phone numbers of tradesmen to call for estimates.

It will also improve your fat distribution and lead to a bit more muscle (although a lot of that gain depends on your lifestyle choices, too, so if you sit on your arse eating pork rinds and fries, it's unlikely all the testosterone in Toledo would give you an ounce of new muscle or less fat around the equator). TRT may also, of course, improve some of those PADAM symptoms listed earlier.

On the downside, there's the inevitable set of side effects and complications that might arise from taking testosterone, such as:

- unfavourable changes in HDL cholesterol and triglyceride levels (although, as stated earlier, studies done so far indicate that the overall effect of TRT on cardiovascular health seems to be either neutral or slightly beneficial)
- a lower sperm count
- an increase in the volume of red blood cells (polycythemia)
- acne
- liver abnormalities (this has been limited to some oral preparations)
- testicular atrophy (usually a problem in younger men who, as my son would aver, have bigger balls than old guys and more room for shrinkage)
- breast growth
- mood swings
- behaviour changes
- fluid retention
- worsening of sleep apnea

To be fair, these are relatively infrequent and generally tolerable side effects, but they can happen, and if millions more men were to take TRT, I am sure we would see a rise in these problems and complaints.

Bottom line, guys: for now, I remain unconvinced of the need to take any hormones as we get older. A bit more memory loss, however, and I might change my mind—if there's any of it left to change, that is.

{4}

THE PROSTATE—OR THE TERMINATOR, BECAUSE IT GETS ALL MEN IN THE END

• • •

The dog and the human are the only two mammals whose prostates give them trouble. Could that be because they're also the most domesticated animals?

DR. MARTIN GLEAVE, urologist

I have three standard speeches in my public-speaking repertoire, each of which has been given a fond nickname by members of my family. The speech I give most often describes strategies for adopting a healthier lifestyle, a speech I call "Healthy Lifestyle—Myth or Reality?" My son Tim, who once heard me give this talk three times in one week, calls it the "s.o.s." speech, "because," he told me after sitting through the third rendition, "it's the same old shit every time, Dad." That boy has a career as a lawyer in front of him, I think, or perhaps as an editorial writer. The second speech I often give carries the title "Menopause—The Best Years." My wife, however, a woman of a certain age, has dubbed this speech "Menopause—Or Hey! Turn the Bloody Heat Down, I'm Boiling Here." And finally, there is my favourite and most requested talk, the one that I call "The Prostate—An Owner's Manual" and that my wife has renamed "The Terminator, Because It Gets All Men in the End."

I hate to say this but she's dead right. The prostate does indeed get every man in the end. The prostate is the "ha-ha, you're it" gland, the gender leveller, the even-upper, that little-but-not-little-enough gland that squarely pays us men back for all those years during which we wondered and frequently scoffed at our partner's and female friends' often relentless struggles with periods, pregnancies, PMS, postpartum pits, and all those other hormonal and glandular changes to which women are biologically captive.

As the years go by, however, it is practically inevitable that the prostate will force itself into an aging man's unwilling consciousness, and pay him back for all that scoffing, so that for far too many a man, the prostate eventually becomes the body part he mournfully rues the most as he stands sleepily, for the second or third time that night, jiggling in that Hebraic shaking-prayer stance in front of his toilet at five A.M., having been jolted awake yet again by pressure from his bladder, waiting impatiently for that weak yellow ribbon to begin its slow trickle down (but not necessarily straight down), and ruefully recalling a time he could go without going for over ten hours, and when he could still hit a tree or a zucchini plant from a distance of at least five yards. Now he can hardly hit the toilet bowl that lies immediately below him, a fact that his partner and the telltale dried-up spots on the bathroom floor regularly remind him of.

What Is a Prostate and Where Can You Find One?

The prostate is a small gland that's part of the male genitourinary system, the name doctors apply to—what else—the combination of urinary and genital systems. When a man is young, the prostate is not big, and is invariably described as walnut-sized or the size of a large strawberry, certainly not large at all when compared with organs such as the liver and spleen. Even when it grows or enlarges, a process called benign hyperplasia, the prostate doesn't become much bigger than a large apricot. Doctors, by the way, as I'm sure you've noticed, are the most imagination-challenged people on earth so the only things we ever compare organs or tissues to are fruits and veggies and the occasional nut.

Now the reason it's important to explain how large a prostate may become is that if the prostate were merely an average body part, size wouldn't matter, just as size doesn't really matter for the other important parts of a male's sexual apparatus. ("Such as his brain," my wife suggests. Right again. For a bookseller, that woman sure knows her anatomy.) For the prostate, however, as for a semidetached bungalow and a small business, the only things that really matter are location, location, location. So it's where the prostate has chosen to set up shop that makes it such a problem-filled gland. The prostate, you see, is located directly below the bladder and in front of the rectum, where it just happens to surround the urethra, the tube through which urine and semen must pass on their way to the breathlessly awaiting world.

This location leads to two problems. The first and more minor of these is that a prostate cannot be felt through the thick abdominal wall, which is thicker in some men than in others, of course. That means that the only way to palpate the prostate is to put a finger (yes, it's only one finger, guys; it just feels like five) into the rectum and push up. This is called a digital rectal exam, or DRE (most aging men think that DRE actually stands for dreaded rectal exam, and younger ones think it's for that rap star, Dr. Dre, but hey, they'll learn better one day, ha, ha, ha), a procedure that most men look forward to about as much as they look forward to an excursion with the wife to buy new shoes. (A cute *New Yorker* cartoon: two husbands leashed side by side to topped-up parking meters in front of Bloomingdale's. Been there, by the way, and certainly felt like that.)

The second problem with the prostate's location is more serious and disturbing: when the prostate grows, it squeezes the urethra, with the consequences I shall describe below.

Do You Really Need a Prostate?

The short answer is no. After all, women do just fine without one. Men do need a prostate, however, if they want to procreate the natural way—that is, without the assistance of an in vitro clinic that can pass on your DNA without your active participation.

So what does the prostate do? It helps sperm survive. You see, seminal fluid originates in the testicles, and from there it has to take a sort of sperm portage by first passing upwards through the vas deferens. From the vas, the seminal fluid passes into the prostate via structures called ejaculatory ducts. Ejaculatory ducts are a sort of way station, where seminal fluid can lay-by for a while before being ejected into the urethra, and finally to, well, that depends on which way you're leaning at the time.

The problem with this setup is that sperm cells are not very large guys, and to a sperm cell, that long transpenile voyage is a very trying and arduous journey. So it's not surprising that they require a rejuvenation hit on their trip. The prostate gland (along with the seminal vesicles that connect to the ejaculatory ducts) serves as the Sperm City Café, so when the seminal fluid passes through, Flo and the rest of the café's waitresses top it up with added liquid as well as nutrients to help the sperm on their suicide mission.

How Your Prostate Can Change Your Life

The three most common prostate conditions are:

- infection or inflammation (prostatitis)
- benign prostatic growth (hyperplasia)
- prostate cancer

Prostatitis

Until the age of forty or so, most men can safely ignore their prostates, and nearly all of us are only too happy to do so. The exceptions are those guys unlucky enough to develop a prostate inflammation or infection, both of which are called prostatitis. The difference between an inflammation and an infection is that with an infection, a recognizable infectious agent accounts for the symptoms, although as many men have found out to their chagrin, often that agent, like a teenager who has chores to do, cannot be easily located or isolated. With a prostate inflammation, no known infectious agent can be detected, although the process may have started as an infection and the responsible party has now fled the scene, like that broker who assured me that those Enron shares would go up, up, up. The shares didn't go up but he sure did—to Antigua, to the Caymans, to Bermuda, and to many other hot spots where he flew on my money.

Acute Bacterial Prostatitis Acute bacterial prostate infections are, happily, relatively infrequent events. This infection tends to happen mainly in young men and older men with large prostates. Acute prostatitis often explodes with many of the sudden severe symptoms that women who have had a bladder infection will instantly recognize: a burning sensation when urinating, a need to urinate often, a need to urinate NOW THIS MINUTE, and for some men the worst symptom—when they get there, they just can't go as easily as is their wont. Other symptoms include fever, pain in either the low back or the low abdomen, chills, and a general feeling of sickness, what my son Jonah, the MBA problem solver and Powerpoint presenter, rather accurately calls, "feeling like shit." Well, he's an MBA, not a doctor. We doctors are more scientific so we would say "feeling like feces."

A bacterial infection leaves the prostate swollen and inflamed, so that when it's palpated it is tender and "boggy." Treatment of acute prostatitis involves using antibiotics in high enough doses to kill all the little buggers. Usually that means taking a lot of antibiotic, because if you think of the prostate as a bacterial spa, warm and wet and well supplied with life-sustaining liquids, nutrients, and other bacteria to consort with, it is clear that the bacteria must be hit regularly and very hard if they are to be ousted. This usually means taking antibiotics for a month and sometimes longer.

Chronic Bacterial Prostatitis Chronic bacterial prostatitis is a real pain in the butt for everyone who has to deal with it, although it's clearly more of a pain for the patient than the doctor. A chronic bacterial prostate infection is produced by an acute infection that no longer responds to short-term use of antibiotics. Symptoms may include pain in the low back or low abdomen, as well as the need to void urgently, frequency of urination, burning on urination, and—here's the real kicker—pain on ejaculation.

But sadly, it often gets even worse than that. What can possibly be worse than pain on ejaculation, you ask? To diagnose the infection, the physician usually opts to get a sample of fluid from the prostate, and he does this via a prostatic massage, the kind of procedure that makes every man who gets one feel convinced that he's going steady with the doctor afterwards. Also, like an unemployed house-guest brother-in-law, chronic bacterial infections of the prostate are hard to get rid of. Treatment consists of several weeks and often months of antibiotics, and unfortunately, the antibiotic regimen must often be repeated since this problem has a habit of recurring. Some men cannot come off the antibiotic at all because their symptoms recur as soon as they discontinue their medication.

Nonbacterial Prostatitis If you are going to feel sorry for anyone, guys, save your pity for the bro who develops nonbacterial prostatitis. Not only is this a visitor who comes to stay, but as with that stray alley cat that came by for only one evening, two tops, and who has now become an unremovable statue on your living room couch, there is also not a whole lot you can do to get rid of nonbacterial prostatitis when it lodges chez vous.

The symptoms of nonbacterial prostatitis are the same as for bacterial prostatitis. A whole host of possible suspects, such as *Chlamydia trachomatis* and *Mycoplasma hominis,* have been linked with a higher risk of nonbacterial prostatitis, but these organisms are also found in the urethras of males without this condition, so something else must be going on in guys who end up with nonbacterial prostatitis besides simple exposure to potentially infective organisms.

If doctors don't know what causes nonbacterial prostatitis, how do they treat it? Well, not knowing the cause of a condition has never stopped doctors from rushing in to treat it, and so it is with this baby as well. It is usually treated with antibiotics directed at the organisms that might be culpable, such as those nasty chlamydiae. Other modes of therapy that have been tried include regular prostatic massage (although I don't think you need a certified massage therapist for this), ultrasound, hot baths, and muscle relaxants. Relaxation therapy, biofeedback, and counselling have also been tried because of the observation that men with this problem are worriers (well, you would worry, too, I think, if you had a persistent pain in your butt that doctors couldn't get rid of). Men with this condition are also advised to avoid biking and horseback riding (I leave it to your imagination to figure out why) as well as to avoid or at least decrease their intake of substances known to make prostate symptoms worse. These include aspartame, caffeine, spicy foods, and alcohol, but as a long-time lover of coffee, pickles, chilis, wine, and Diet Coke, five of the seven essential food groups (salami and garlic are the others), I must say that if these substances do not obviously make your symptoms worse, there is no real reason to avoid them entirely.

Also, as every person with this condition invariably asks: "So what about *it*, eh, Doc?" Good news, guys. *It* is OK. In fact, these days most specialists say that "it" should be mandatory on the theory that just as an old car needs an oil change from time to time, the prostate needs its fluids emptied regularly too, and happily you are supposed to empty your gland considerably more often than you change the oil in your car. But please don't ask me how often. Whatever you believe is fine by me, unless, that is, you start going blind or your hands start shaking. That's probably too often.

Finally, the only good thing to say about all prostate infections is that none of them has been linked to a higher risk of prostate cancer, although I'm sure that particular worry keeps a lot of men with nonbacterial prostatitis up at night.

Benign Prostatic Hyperplasia—Why Does It Take You So Long to Pee, Dad?

The prostate grows with age in every man. And grows. And grows. A man who lives to age sixty has a 50 per cent chance of suffering symptoms from an enlarged prostate, or benign prostatic hyperplasia (but 50 per cent of men still don't), and if he is lucky enough to live into his mid-eighties, he has a 90 per cent chance of suffering from an enlarged prostate (but again, we see a lucky 10 per cent of centenarians who don't have prostate problems; I just hope they're alert enough to appreciate their good luck). So your prostate will grow, guy, but what is vital to underline is this: the prostate grows at different rates in different men, and it causes symptoms at different prostate volumes in different men. And it's the symptoms that should concern us most, not the size of the gland. Yes, once again, size doesn't matter, although if you have a grapefruit-sized prostate, I'd worry about it even if it isn't causing symptoms.

Why do I make such an issue of distinguishing between prostate size and prostate symptoms? Because many enlarged prostates do not require treatment. It's only when an enlarged prostate causes symptoms significant enough to interfere with its owner's life or when it grows large enough to produce potentially significant medical complications such as infections that its owner requires therapy. The common estimate is that one in four men require treatment for benign prostatic hyperplasia (BPH) by the age of eighty, but that also means that three in four do not, something to comfort you tonight on your second postmidnight voiding expedition.

Why the prostate grows is not clear. Hormones, especially testosterone, must play a key role, but most studies have been unable to find a consistent link between testosterone levels and prostate size, perhaps because testosterone exerts its greatest effect on the prostate very early in life. Most experts also believe that environmental influences must play a role in making the prostate swell, although again, studies have failed to nail down consistent patterns between environmental factors and prostate size.

Symptoms ***Prostatism*** refers to the complex of symptoms produced by an enlarged prostate, which include most prominently:

- having to get up at night to urinate, sometimes several times
- a slower and weaker urine flow
- a feeling that the bladder has not been completely emptied after urinating
- a need to urinate more often
- a sense of urgency, so that when you gotta go, you really gotta go
- dribbling, although this is clearly not the same kind of dribbling you associate with Michael Jordan, but it is the kind of dribbling every woman can appreciate (although I'm not sure "appreciate" is the best term to use here)
- blood in the urine, which may only be detectable on a urinalysis
- sexual dysfunction

The American Urological Association grades most of these symptoms on a scale from one (mild) to five (will-no-one-rid-me-of-this-gland?), and the higher the overall score, the more likely it is that therapy will offer some relief.

Do not, however, assume that if you develop the symptoms listed above, you are merely suffering from benign prostatic hyperplasia, and that you can ignore it until you choose to visit the doctor, oh, sometime in 2009. Rather, you must see your doctor pretty quickly to ensure that these symptoms are not the first sign of prostate cancer, a prostate infection, or even a non-urological problem, all of which can produce similar symptoms. (To be accurate, you don't actually "see" the doctor while he or she is checking your prostate, but if you do, the Cirque du Soleil would like to give you an audition.) For example, some men who complain about having to get up at night to pee are not suffering from benign prostatic hyperplasia but rather from some type of sleep disturbance, such as sleep apnea (see Chapter 7), and they only get up so often to pee because of that sleep problem. In other words, although the cart may be the need to urinate, the horse is actually the sleep disorder.

Is there any reason to treat benign prostatic hyperplasia that is not causing significant symptoms? Not really. First, there does not seem to be any link between BPH and prostate cancer (although they often do occur in the same elderly gent, of course, but not because one led to the other). Second, although the occasional large prostate can suddenly cause complications that require urgent medical intervention, such as an inability to urinate or recurrent bladder infections, these complications don't commonly occur without significant symptoms. As stated earlier, for the vast majority of men who possess a larger prostate, it's not the size but the symptoms that determine the need for therapy, and even a large prostate does not require surgery if the symptoms remain mild. And the good news is that the symptoms do not have to progress relentlessly. For example, one study found that over four years of observation, the majority of patients with mild symptoms of benign prostatic hyperplasia did not go on to suffer severe symptoms. Another study compared men who opted for early surgery with men who chose watchful waiting for their benign prostatic hyperplasia (the doctor was watchful, the patient was waiting) and found that only 24 per cent of the latter group required surgery over the seven years of the study.

Treatment Lifestyle interventions, particularly diet and exercise, are not known to make any difference to how much or how rapidly a prostate will grow, nor does the rate of ejaculation, although for obvious reasons, most guys will choose to believe that the more it's emptied, the healthier the gland.

For active treatment, the herb saw palmetto is widely used in Europe for benign prostatic hyperplasia and is commonly said to relieve symptoms Over There. The objective data is mixed, however, so that while some small studies have indicated that saw palmetto might help relieve symptoms and slow prostatic growth, others (including a recent large trial) have found no benefit.

I am of the age where I need something to relieve symptoms, however, and as I predicted when I first wrote *Midlife Man,* I am indeed sawing the palmetto. I have no idea if it's working, but I just love swallowing those huge capsules.

Finasteride and dutasteride, drugs known as 5-alpha reductase inhibitors, can help slow the progression of benign prostatic hyperplasia and quell symptoms by slowing down the breakdown of testosterone to its more active metabolites. As well, several other drugs known as alpha blockers (terazosin, prazosin, doxazosin, and others) are also effective in reducing the symptoms of benign prostatic hyperplasia by relaxing muscle fibres in the prostate (I bet you never knew you had muscles down there). These latter drugs don't slow the growth of the prostate. Rather they improve symptoms associated with an enlarged gland, such as the need to urinate at night or the feeling that the bladder is not completely emptied after urinating. They can also improve what urologists refer to as "peak flow rate," meaning that the tiny tinny trickle through a tense and thickened prostate is somewhat enhanced.

It's important to note, though, that in many studies, placebos have worked nearly as well as the expensive drugs have, and placebos have even produced side effects not unlike those produced by the medications. Placebos work so well, in fact, that in one study the men who had been on them still claimed an improvement in their symptoms two years after the study had stopped, and they refused to give up the placebos when the study had ended and they were told that the pills contained nothing but sugar. Now these are guys I would love to talk to about my Enron shares.

If you do decide to go on treatment, it's always best to start with only one drug because that minimizes the risk of side effects, although an intriguing study has concluded that the combination of a 5-alpha reductase inhibitor and an alpha blocker works better than either drug alone.

Among the side effects to be expected on finasteride and dutasteride, decreased libido and impotence stand out, as they usually do, whereas dizziness is often the main problem with alpha blockers—not too surprising when you learn that these drugs are also useful in lowering blood pressure.

Also, a recent study found that injecting Botox into the prostate could improve BPH symptoms, and as an added benefit, the urologist also got rid of any wrinkles he found there.

When your troublesome symptoms do not respond to medication, you must turn to surgery for relief, and here there are several choices with several more in the works. In fact, you can think of a urologist's office as a kind of Shopping Channel, where you get more choices to purchase something you don't really want than you had ever imagined possible. The old standby for prostate surgery is usually referred to rather unkindly but not inaccurately as a Roto-Rooter job, although the official term is transurethral resection of the prostate, or TURP. In this procedure, the surgeon pushes his instruments into the prostate via the urethra and then hacks away. At least, that's the way most patients view a TURP, although to be fair, urologists see it somewhat more benignly—but then they have a better, and less painful, seat in the stands to view it from.

As a potential improvement on the old hack-and-slash method, some surgeons burn the tissue with an electric current or a laser, or they—hold on to your seats, guys—microwave the tissue with a gadget called a Prostatron during transurethral microwave thermotherapy, or TUMT, although if I were having this done on me, I would want strict guarantees that the instrument would not start any arcing in there. Another technique is a procedure known as transurethral needle ablation, or TUNA, in which a catheter with electrodes attached to its end is inserted into the prostate via the urethra. With the catheter in place, the urologist lets loose radio waves of a specific frequency, which not only kill the tissue around the electrodes but, if you're really lucky, pick up the Rush Limbaugh show at the same time. Well, better that than country-and-western music.

Prostate Cancer

What do Robert Goulet, Arnold Palmer, Bob Dole, Colin Powell, John Kerry, and General Norman Schwartzkopf have in common? Yes, they are all has-beens, but the other link between them is that they all also have prostate cancer, as do Nelson Mandela, Joe Torre, Sean Connery, and Robert de Niro, so you don't have to be quite past it to end up with prostate cancer—although it helps. Prostate cancer is an equal-opportunity cancer that can strike any man, and it strikes a lot of men.

How many? Well, everyone knows that women have a one-in-nine chance of getting breast cancer if they live long enough. But how many of you know that as men we have a one-in-six chance of being diagnosed with prostate cancer during our lifetimes, and that 3 per cent of us will eventually die from that malignancy? After skin cancer, prostate cancer is the most common cancer affecting men in the developed world and, after lung cancer, prostate cancer is the second leading cause of deaths from cancer in men in the developed world. Currently, over twenty thousand men a year are diagnosed with prostate cancer in Canada, a number that's growing rapidly because of better tests, because of a huge growth in the number of frightened men like me who have run off to get themselves tested for prostate cancer, and most of all because of increased life expectancy in men, since the longer a man lives, the higher his risk of prostate cancer. Happily, though, over 90 per cent of prostate cancers remain dormant, so that most men die *with* prostate cancer and not *of* prostate cancer (see below).

Risk Factors What do researchers know about the risk factors for prostate cancer? Lots, but not nearly enough.

For most men, age is by far the most important risk factor. Prostate cancer affects only about one in thirteen thousand men at age forty, but after that the older we get, the higher our risk, so that one in six men over the age of seventy will be diagnosed with prostate cancer. Race too plays an important role so that African American men have twice the risk of North Americans of European descent.

About 9 to 10 per cent of all prostate cancers are estimated to be caused by genetic predisposition. Thus, a man who has a first-degree male relative (father, brother, grandfather) who has had prostate cancer is two to three times as likely as his peers to develop prostate cancer himself, and the younger the relative was when he developed the cancer, the higher this man's risk. A man with two first-degree relatives who had prostate cancer has an eightfold to tenfold increased risk himself. Familial prostate cancers also tend to occur more frequently in younger men, and they also tend to be more aggressive cancers.

A man's risk of prostate cancer also goes up if his mother's family has a strong history of this tumour, and just to scare you even more, there may also be a slight increase in colon and breast cancers in such families.

Prostate cancer cells need testosterone to grow but the relationship between testosterone and prostate cancer is much like the one between my mother and me—much more complicated than it seems on the surface. Thus, some studies have linked higher rates of prostate cancer to higher levels of testosterone and free testosterone, although others, like the authoritative Massachusetts Male Aging Study, did not find such a link. Moreover, a study from Duke University found that men with small shoulder spans in relation to the rest of their bodies—someone like yours truly who has been described as shoulder challenged, and that's by my trainer, no less, although as I answered him with a smirk, "Better that than brain-challenged, eh?" to which he said, "Huh?"—also seem to have a higher risk of prostate cancer. Walking around with your chest puffed out and your shoulders held back as far as they'll go will not change your risk of prostate cancer, however, because what this study really indicates is that the influence that testosterone exerts on your risk of prostate cancer may be set very early in life—your shoulder span is determined before you're born—and so measuring testosterone levels later in life may not reflect testosterone's real effects on the prostate.

Another potential risk factor for prostate cancer that has long intrigued researchers is an interruption to the flow of sperm, such as from a vasectomy, and a few years ago a highly publicized study did indeed claim to have discovered a link between vasectomies at a young age (under thirty-five) and an increased risk of prostate cancer. Most other studies have failed to confirm this link, however, and the current consensus is that even if a vasectomy does raise the risk of prostate cancer, that increase is very negligible (although for most men, a "negligible increased risk" is an oxymoron when it comes to genital-area cancers). In any case, the benefits of a vasectomy far outweigh the slight possibility of an increased risk for prostate cancer.

Environmental and dietary factors play a large role on how prostate cancer can affect you, so although microscopic evidence for the presence of prostate cancer cells is fairly constant in men throughout the world, the rates at which prostate cancers grow to cause trouble vary significantly in different areas of the world. For example, Chinese men living in China have among the lowest rates of death from prostate cancer in the world. But when Chinese men move to North America, their risk of death from prostate cancer goes up, and within two generations the rates for their offspring are much closer to those for other men born in North America. To give even more credence to an environmental role in prostate cancer development, prostate cancer rates are gradually rising in all those countries that are steadily becoming more westernized. So along with the SUVs and the fridges and the TVs that Chinese men in Beijing are accumulating in such huge numbers, they will probably also soon inherit the same rate of prostate cancer that their North American brothers have long had to themselves.

So, of all the most significant westernizing influences—drugs, sex, Madonna videos, and bowling—which ones, do you think, are most responsible for this rising tide of prostate cancers? As always, heavy drinking, smoking, and obesity have been related to this cancer, although the guiltiest party is probably our western diet. But what in the diet hurts the prostate and what helps the prostate are still a matter of much debate.

We do know, for example, that a typical North American diet low in fibre, low in fruits and veggies, and most important, high in fat, especially saturated fat derived from red meat and dairy products, has been correlated with a higher risk of prostate cancer and a worsening of an already existing malignancy as well. So has, interestingly, a diet higher in polyunsaturated fats such as those derived from some vegetable oils. Another intriguing dietary risk might be calcium. In the Health Professionals' Follow-Up Study, a high daily calcium intake (from dairy products mostly) was correlated with a 4.6 times higher rate of prostate cancer. Rather than saying this was the fault of the saturated fats in the dairy products, the study authors laid the blame squarely on the calcium.

Some healthy foods and elements that have been linked with lower rates of prostate disease include:

- cruciferous veggies, such as cauliflower and broccoli
- high-fibre foods such as whole grain cereals, seeds, and nuts
- monounsaturated fats such as those found in nuts, seeds, and some vegetables
- green tea
- omega-3 fatty acids and fish oils
- soy products (although this is supported by studies in animals, not humans)
- red wine

Regarding this last item, everybody is always pleased to learn that regular intake of moderate amounts of red wine has been linked with an up to 50 per cent lower risk of prostate cancer, especially of the most aggressive tumours. You should keep in mind, though, that binge drinking has been linked with higher risks.

One of the most intriguing links between diet and prostate cancer suggests the risk of prostate cancer is lowered by a high intake of lycopene, an antioxidant in the carotene family. Lycopene is found in large amounts in watermelon, red grapefruit, and some shellfish, but by far the largest amounts are in tomatoes, especially cooked tomatoes, because cooking the tomatoes breaks down the lycopene and allows it to be more easily absorbed. And boy are cooked tomatoes ever good for the back end! Thus, in a famous study of health professionals, three of the four foods found to be associated most strongly with a lower risk of prostate cancer were tomato sauce, tomatoes, and pizza, although I must say that I am just a tad suspicious when a study headed by a man with an Italian surname finds that we would all be better off if we ate more tomato sauce and pizza. By the way, despite what that famous pizza expert, my son, Tim, has to say, this does not really mean that the healthiest diet a young man can eat to protect his heart, his skeleton, and his prostate includes nachos (for the cheese, of course), salsa (for the lycopene), and beer (for the antioxidants). Where does he come up with these ideas?

Besides lycopene, other vitamins and minerals that may play a large role in preventing prostate cancer include:

- Vitamin E. Studies have indicated that men, even men who smoke, who take daily supplements of vitamin E might reduce their risk of prostate cancer by as much as 30 per cent and their risk of dying from prostate cancer by over 40 per cent, although this is still a matter of much debate, and several ongoing studies are trying to determine if taking large supplemental doses of vitamin E can indeed lower the risk of prostate cancer.
- Beta-carotene. A study of fifteen thousand Harvard doctors found that those who had the highest blood levels of beta-carotene had the lowest rates of prostate cancer, although large intake of vitamin A has been linked to poorer bone health, so this is one I would leave alone for now.
- Vitamin D. This one appears to be the best of the lot. It is known, for a start, that in northern countries, where people have less exposure to sunlight than in other parts of the world (sunlight promotes the body's production of vitamin D), men have higher rates of prostate cancer. Further, a recent study found that men with higher blood levels of vitamin D (both from sunshine and from dietary and supplemental sources) had a 50 per cent lower risk of developing prostate cancer than men with lower vitamin D levels.
- Folic acid. Some researchers believe that a deficiency in folic acid may also be a potential risk factor for prostate cancer, although a recent study found that people who supplement with folic acid develop dementia at a faster rate than those who don't, and you don't really want to spare your behind while you fry your brain, do you?

- Selenium. This is another one getting lots of interest because of a study that found that men taking selenium supplements had a significantly lowered risk of prostate cancer.
- Boron. A much touted study found that a high intake of boron, which happily is found in red grapes, red wine, nuts, apples, watermelon, dried fruits, and even chocolate, is related to a lower risk of prostate cancer, and even if it doesn't prevent that malignancy, you'll die happier if you've eaten lots of boron-contaning foods, believe me.
- Turmeric. Curcurmin, which is better known as turmeric, and which is the stuff that gives curry its colour, is also said to inhibit the growth of prostate cancer cells, although the bad news is that it turns your prostate yellow—just kidding!.

Bottom line? Same old, same old. When trying to prevent prostate cancer, you should eat what you'd eat to try to prevent all chronic diseases: more grains, fibre, fruits, and veggies (especially cooked tomatoes), and you might want to use some curry or mustard to flavour it up. You should also eat less red meat and less saturated and trans fats. And it never hurts to exercise, either.

One other "environmental" factor is the use of ASA and other nonsteroidal anti-inflammatories, which may play a protective role against this cancer.

Finally, to keep you reading this far, I've left the factor you have all no doubt been waiting for to the end: intercourse, or more accurately, ejaculation, because as we all know and as our mothers warned us, most ejaculation is not done as part of a sexual act with others. Feh! So what effect does frequent intercourse or, if you're unlucky or just not handy, infrequent ejaculation have on your risk of prostate cancer?

Well, clap your hands, boys, if they're not shaking, because the news here is good. Although one older well-designed study that, needless to say, garnered a lot of headlines—and fear—found that men who have more frequent intercourse have a higher risk of prostate cancer, a much better recent study found that frequent ejaculation actually protects against prostate cancer. Some have even tried to pin a number on it (in case you want to do some homework) and have come up with this: more than twelve ejaculations per month starts to confer some benefit, and the more the better. Woo hoo! Woo hoo!

But why the different results from two equally reputable studies? you may well ask. It's all to do with definition. You see, even if you show that men who have more intercourse (or at least who claim to have more) end up with more prostate cancer, that does not establish a cause-and-effect relationship between frequency of intercourse and prostate cancer. It may just be that the hormones (and other factors) that drive certain men to adopt a philosophy of "Damn the torpedoes! I've got to empty my load, no matter what the consequences!" may also be what condemns such men to a higher risk of prostate cancer. More probably, according to recent data, the more sexual partners a man has over his lifetime, the higher his risk of STDs, and it's pretty certain now that the more STDs a man suffers in his life, the more likely he is to develop prostate cancer. Thus, studies have linked high rates of gonorrhea, chlamydia infections, and papilloma virus infections with higher rates of prostate cancer. So if you're practising safe sex, and if you're not, you bloody well should be, there is no evidence that slowing down the rate at which you empty that old sac of sperm will lower your risk of prostate cancer, so full steam ahead, boys, and may God be with you.

One other preventive strategy against prostate cancer that I must address is the use of drugs. First, a much ballyhooed recent study found that the risk of prostate cancer can be lowered in a high-risk individual by about 25 per cent if he takes either finasteride or dutasteride prophylactially. Three caveats for this finasteride-free-for-all, though: 1) there's still no proof that this treatment actually extends life expectancy, 2) we have absolutely no idea what such an approach would do to or for normal-risk guys, and 3) the guys who ended up with prostate cancer while taking finasteride seemed to develop a fairly aggressive form of the disease.

Then, there's the ubiquitous use of nonsteroidal anti-inflammatories (NSAIDs), including ASA (see Chapter 5), which several studies have linked to lower rates of several cancers, including prostate cancer. But since no good study has proved that taking an NSAID will actually prevent cancer, and since NSAIDs have several potential drawbacks, it seems to me that no man should be taking ASA or any NSAID for the sole purpose of nurturing his prostate. If you're taking an NSAID or ASA for any other reason, however, the good news is that it might also be protecting your prostate.

One last and very important note: although I, along with most other middle-aged guys, tend to make a lot of bad jokes about prostate disease and prostate cancer, in large part because it is not yet a part of our lives, prostate cancer is not a laughing matter. Instead, all too frequently it's a source of a great deal of stress and depression. In fact, men diagnosed with prostate cancer are more likely to commit suicide than men diagnosed with any other kind of cancer, and several studies have shown that a man diagnosed with prostate cancer will do much better if he involves his wife or partner in his decision making and care.

Symptoms Unfortunately, in its most curable stage, when a tumour is still small and confined to the prostate, prostate cancer does not generally produce any symptoms to announce its presence. If you remember nothing else from this chapter, remember this: prostate cancer is a silent killer.

As a prostate cancer grows, it can cause symptoms similar to those associated with benign prostatic hyperplasia, and when it spreads, it will produce symptoms associated with the area it invades. For example, if it metastasizes to a bone, a favourite place for prostate cancer to spread to, it will cause severe pain associated with bone cancer.

Diagnosis Prostate cancer is often compared with breast cancer—both cancers increase significantly with age; both are hormonally driven cancers; breast cancer is the second leading cause of death from cancer in women, while prostate cancer is the second leading cause of death from cancer in men; and until recently, both cancers had been neglected for far too long by research funding agencies. But these two cancers differ in at least one vital respect: you don't ever want to diagnose prostate cancer through a self-examination. Rather, in the diagnosis of prostate cancer, you are completely in the hand (it's only one) of a stranger.

Unfortunately, until relatively recently, the only way to diagnose prostate cancer was through a digital rectal exam, what men of a certain vintage like to call the "old one-fingered salute," a procedure that for some strange reason seems to be the butt of much urological humour. It's not unusual, for example, for a urologist to tell a whimpering, butt-up man, "You know, George, I'm not really sure what's going on up there. I think I want a second opinion." And as a joke, he pretends to get another digit ready. (This is an excellent illustration of why urologists rarely get invited to mixed parties, "mixed" meaning that there are other human beings there.)

Although I wouldn't say this to a guy fetalized on the exam table, the digital rectal exam is rather insensitive—that is, it cannot detect small tumours. No surprise, then, that less than 40 per cent of prostate cancers detected by a digital rectal exam are still confined to the prostate, so by the time a prostate cancer is palpable with a digital rectal exam, there is a likelihood that it has already spread. For this reason, the digital rectal exam is a rather poor screening tool for prostate cancer. That is why there has been so much optimism about a blood test for prostate cancer, the first of which is the prostate-specific antigen (PSA) test. For nearly two decades now, it has been hoped that the PSA would become a useful, sensitive, and specific screening test for prostate cancer and would replace the need to do a digital rectal exam. That has still not happened.

PSA is an enzyme produced by prostate cells that liquefies the ejaculate. Small amounts of PSA leak into the circulation and are easily measured, and since PSA is largely specific for prostate cells, the level of PSA in the blood *should* be a good measure of what's going on in the prostate. A "normal" reading has long been declared as anything less than 4.0 ng/mL. But we now know that "normal" is not normal for all men, so that PSA varies with age and prostate volume, meaning that a normal PSA level for a younger man is closer to 2.0 ng/mL, while a normal PSA for an older man with a large prostate may be above 5.0 or even 6.0. Also, men at higher risk for prostate cancer should be concerned with any level of PSA above 2.0, especially if the PSA is increasing year-to-year. Thus, a PSA level of even 4.0 would be significant in a man who had a reading of 0.5 two years ago and 1.5 one year ago.

Unfortunately, PSA levels are not nearly as specific for prostate cancer as we would like them to be, primarily because PSA levels can go up with just about anything that affects the prostate, not just cancer (PSA is also secreted in very small amounts by other tissues). Thus, the PSA level goes up after ejaculation (you have to avoid ejaculating for forty-eight hours before getting tested, not as harsh a requirement as most middle-aged guys would like you to believe it is). PSA also increases with benign prostatic hyperplasia, following a vigorous prostate massage, and occasionally after exercise. It can even go up following the dreaded digital derrière dilatation. So one slightly high measure usually means nothing. A level that continues to rise is more likely to be significant, and then again, it might not. It all depends, you see—although we're not completely sure yet what it depends on. We do know, however, that a large majority of men with PSA levels between 4.0 and 10.0 ng/mL (which is considered high) do not have a malignancy. This is known as a false-positive result, that is, a test result that's elevated indicating the presence of a particular disease we're trying to detect, but when that person is investigated with better tests, that disease is not detected. And there's the rub because based on the widely accepted axiom—one held in equal esteem by both a terrified patient and a malpractice-phobic physician—that all abnormal test results must be explained (or else!), a man with an elevated PSA level will nearly always undergo further tests to rule out prostate cancer.

This is a real problem because these tests involve ultrasound of the prostate (that's not too bad) as well as multiple biopsies (that can be bad). Not only is this an emotionally traumatic situation for most men—if you think the average guy feels ridiculously sorry for himself when he has a cold, wait till you see the same guy after he's been told someone is going to stick a needle up his arse and may find something that could eventually leave him impotent and incontinent—but these are also costly and potentially hazardous procedures. Although a prostate biopsy is often referred to as a "minor" procedure, it's always wise to remember that most doctors' definition of a minor procedure is "something that's done on someone else." Even minor procedures can occasionally result in complications such as excess bleeding and infection and, rarely, neurological damage.

An added problem with prostate biopsies is that they're not always spot on—that is, some cancers are entirely missed when the surgeon aims his needles into the prostate (one study found that roughly one in four cancers is missed on the first attempt at biopsy in men with elevated PSA levels), and even when a lump does yield a biopsy specimen (as most do), there can be disagreement among pathologists as to the significance of the cellular changes. In other words, "cancer" is occasionally in the eye of the beholder.

Of equal concern is the fact that we don't even know what to do with many proven prostate cancers. In other words, even if we detect a prostate cancer through biopsy, we are simply not very good at telling which one of those cancers must be treated because it will inevitably go on to enlarge and spread, and which can safely be left alone because it will grow too slowly to affect that man's life.

Then there is the concern about false-negative results—that is, the test result is normal yet the disease we're looking for is present. Thus, a recent study found that a high percentage of men with prostate cancer (15 per cent, perhaps as high as 25 per cent) had PSA levels deemed to be normal.

It's all enough to shake a boy's confidence in the system, ain't it?

So although there is widespread acceptance of the PSA test as a good measure of followup after cancer therapy (the PSA level should drop into the normal range, and one should worry if it starts to go up again), there is still a lot of controversy about using the PSA by itself as a mass screening test on many millions of men who are healthy and have no reason to suspect they may be harbouring a malignancy, and most of whom will not have prostate cancer even with a raised PSA level. Although most urologists argue that the small risk inherent in extra testing is far outweighed by the benefits of finding all those extra cancers at a still treatable stage, a lot of number crunchers don't agree. In fact, one widely cited recent review concluded that the benefits of PSA as a screening test are still unproven, and that the risks outweigh the benefits.

Interestingly, that's how it was seven years ago when I wrote the first edition of *Midlife Man* and that's how it still is, despite the research that's gone into refining the PSA test and finding alternative tests and more advanced techniques, such as measuring "free" or unbound PSA levels or complexed PSA or PSA velocity or Pro-PSA and several others. The bottom line is that urologists nearly uniformly believe that all men at average risk for prostate cancer should be screened with regular PSA tests from the age of fifty on, while many epidemiologists, as well as many funding health care agencies, still believe that PSA screening in low-risk men is not worth the price.

So what to do, eh? As always, I'm afraid, it all depends on you. The more you worry about such things, the more likely you are to say, "I'll risk the consequences of a false-positive or a false-negative result and get my PSA done. Gulp!" Which is exactly what I did. Once. Five years ago. As a world-class neurotic, I really had no choice, especially after I'd read a study from Canada that concluded that PSA screening could lower the death rate from prostate cancer by up to 69 per cent. I really wanted to be in that number.

I haven't been back since. Why? Well, since I'm not any less neurotic, it's certainly not because I fear dying any less than I used to. Hey, I don't think I'll ever be ready for the Malach Hamavet (the Angel of Death, to a WASP, although doesn't it sound way worse in Hebrew, especially if you can't pronounce "Malach" properly?) when She comes to call. It's just that along the way, I have become more convinced that for me the downsides of PSA testing outweigh the benefits the test might confer. But that's just for me. For now. You may be different, and this is one area I can't really help you with, unless you're a younger man at high risk for prostate cancer and then you should certainly get the test, starting at age forty or so.

If despite my example, you do decide to get PSA screening, another key issue for you is how often to repeat it. Some pro-PSA experts advise having a yearly test, but a study in the *Journal of Urology* found that in a male with a PSA level below 2.0 ng/mL, every two years is probably enough.

Treatment Treatment is far too complex an issue to tackle in a book of this kind, but I will discuss that raging controversy you are all no doubt familiar with: does it even pay to treat certain prostate cancers? The background to this debate is that several studies have suggested that in some men, particularly elderly gents with small tumours, doing nothing, the age-old therapy known as "watchful waiting," leads to the same outcome as the best active interventional treatment. On the one hand, two well-publicized studies have found that men with early stage cancers who elect watchful waiting live just as long as men who receive the best therapy. On the other hand, another equally hyped Scandinavian study found that most men with prostate cancer who elected to do nothing eventually died of that cancer, and it's not a pleasant death. We also know that in our culture, watchful waiting is a very uncomfortable choice, both for the patient who is anxious to do something, and for his doctors, who likewise would love to be able to intervene to alter the natural outcome of this illness. Consequently, over 90 per cent of men with a prostate cancer will elect to "do something." But is "doing something, anything" the wisest course? That's another one that's up to you to decide, I'm afraid. My perspective is this. For younger men (those under sixty and perhaps under sixty-five) with prostate cancer, it seems pretty clear to me that something should be done, although what that "something" should be is often a matter of debate. The factors that must be taken into account include:

- the stage of the tumour (a measure of how far the cancer has spread from its nub in the prostate)
- the probable prognosis for the kind of cancer
- the man's age and how much longer he can expect to live
- the man's overall state of health
- the state of the art in the medical locale where the man resides (this may get me kicked out of the next physicians' golf tournament held in my area, which would not be that much of a loss, to be sure, since they never invite me anyway, but some doctors and institutions re simply more adept at these procedures than others)
- what the doctor suggests
- what the man's partner and family think
- what the man feels his life will be like after whatever choice he makes (will incontinence, for example, make his life simply unbearable?)

The treatment choices that confront every man who's diagnosed with prostate cancer include:

- watchful waiting (as noted above)
- radiation therapy
- cryotherapy (freezing of the cells)

- surgery
- hormonal therapy (this is only for advanced cancers and includes, alas, a procedure to eliminate sex hormones, very like the one that was done on my husky Big Louie at a rather tender age and that turned him into the largest, most sedate, male malamute on the continent with the highest-pitched howl)

Each of these options carries its own risks and benefits, and any man confronted with these choices should do a lot of research and then gather his loved ones and discuss the options. You should not go into this alone.

Surgery, still the standard therapy for most prostate cancers, may, unfortunately leave you with those twin devils of incontinence and impotence as friends for life. The reason for these complications is simple: the nerves and muscles that are involved in both bladder control and erectile ability are in intimate contact with the prostate and are often unavoidably injured in prostate surgery. The good news is that the track record for this surgery has gotten better since the introduction of a machine that can help the surgeon avoid slicing the vital nerves involved in maintaining potency. This machine works on the same principle as a metal detector—the closer the machine gets to a nerve, the louder it beeps. Not only that, a really skilled surgeon is also able to find many of the coins that you have lost over your lifetime, although he may have trouble extracting the quarters.

Radiation therapy used to be reserved for inoperable tumours or for men too weak or too ill to withstand surgery. But over the last few years, a technique called brachytherapy that employs seeds or pellets of radioactive material that are left in place in the tumour has been used to great effect. The major advantage of brachytherapy is that it confines most of the effects of radiation to prostate tissue only and thus carries less risk than older forms of radiation. As a result, brachytherapy is now used for many men who have smaller, localized tumours, although there is still some debate about the long-term results.

One of the newer most intriguing areas of therapeutic research is vaccine therapy. Strictly speaking, this is not a true vaccine, since its purpose is to combat an already existing disease. But the principle in this approach is the same as with a vaccine. Researchers take immune cells called dendrites from the cancer patient's blood, multiply those cells in the lab, expose the dendrites to a component of prostate cancer cells so that the altered dendrites can now recognize cancer cells, and inject these new and wise dendrites into the patient, where they "teach" other immune cells how to seek and destroy the cancer cells. It will be years yet before such a vaccine or the highly anticipated gene therapy is widely available, but the good news is that they're making progress, guys.

There is hope on the horizon. It's just that it's still very distant, so in the meantime, get yourself a good pair of binoculars and try to hold on until one of those ships comes in.

{5}

DISPELLING MYTHS ABOUT DISEASE IN MIDDLE AGE

• • •

Don't it always seem to go that
you don't know what you got till it's gone.

JONI MITCHELL, "Big Yellow Taxi"

Over himself, over his own body
and mind, the individual is sovereign.

JOHN STUART MILL

Not quite.

ART HISTER

Earlier I sprung the no doubt surprising fact on you that most middle-aged men are the original happy gang, or as someone near and dear to me put it, the most smug, most self-sufficient, and most self-congratulatory demographic group you could ever imagine. (She's just annoyed that she's not a middle-aged male, that's all.) There is an important exception to this orgy of unalloyed contentment, however—namely, that cohort of middle-aged guys dealing with chronic illnesses. As my mom is wont to point out, over and over and over again, "If you have your health, Arthur, you have everything," and I would take her word on this one, guys, since at last count my mom did indeed seem to have everything. And she's holding on to it very tightly, too.

Happiness often does depend largely on one's state of health, and sadly, middle age is when a still small but growing number of men start dealing with physical or psychological chronic illness, which not only affects their well-being but also limits their life expectancy. To quote from a study in the *British Medical Journal*, "healthy life expectancy is determined by a relatively limited number of chronic conditions that become more common with increasing age." To be fair, the authors of this study were talking about elderly people dealing with problems such as heart disease, osteoporosis, diabetes, strokes, arthritis, neurodegenerative disorders, depression, cancers, visual loss, cataracts, glaucoma, deafness, and a host of equally cheery conditions. But the first signs of many of these illnesses appear in middle age, and although most of us plan for an old age of contentment, sitting by a fireplace, regaling our mates with tales from our youth, this is actually an illusion. Although we never plan on getting sick, unfortunately, most of us will. And we seem to be getting sick at ever-younger ages. Thus, a recent survey of 980 middle-aged adults attending a family practice clinic in Calgary found that 90 per cent of them already had at least one chronic illness, while just under 50 per cent had five or more chronic health problems, which included such significant entities as high blood pressure, arthritis, depression, and heart disease.

What follows is a description of some of the diseases that you might run into or that might be worrying you as you wade ever deeper into middle age. This is not meant to be an all-inclusive list. My purpose is simply to dispel some myths, to alleviate some anxiety, to poke some fun, to add a pearl of wisdom that your other oyster—your family doc—may have missed, to offer my take on controversial aspects of some health issues, and most of all, to focus on prevention rather than treatment.

Alzheimer's Disease

The only reason I mention Alzheimer's disease in a book on middle age is that most baby boomers are terrified that a single instance of misplacing the car keys is the first hint of impending Alzheimer's disease. This is nonsense. A good definition I once heard of Alzheimer's disease is that although we all forget our keys occasionally, people with Alzheimer's disease forget what the keys are for. Yes, Alzheimer's disease is an eventual threat to your health. (In fact, experts have called the impending increase in dementia cases among baby boomers who hit their senior years a "huge wave" and a "looming epidemic." Yikes! That's us!) But with the exception of certain kinds of genetically linked Alzheimer's, this is not a disease of your middle years. By the way, Alzheimer's disease is really only one of several forms of dementia. Thus, dementias can also be caused by multiple small strokes that affect the brain, by one large stroke, by metabolic abnormalities, and by a host of other conditions. That's why when someone is showing signs of dementia, it's important to determine if they are suffering from a reversible type of dementia, such as one due to drugs or to a metabolic change, and further, to see if anything can be done to slow down the progress of that type of dementia.

For the longest time, dementia seemed to be an inevitable consequence of aging, but we now know that it's not. In fact, according to the leaders of a fascinating study called the Religious Orders Study in which several hundred elderly nuns and priests are being followed unto death to determine what they come down with and what they die of, "memory loss is not an inevitable consequence of aging, but rather is usually the consequence of age-related disease," meaning that it might be nearly entirely preventable.

We also know that the seeds of Alzheimer's disease and other dementias are certainly sown in our middle years, and we now have compelling evidence that we can greatly lower our risk of most forms of dementia by simply following healthier lifestyles. For example, a study of more than 8,800 men published in the journal *Neurology* concluded that the risk of dementia in later years is increased substantially if a midlife man:

- smokes
- has diabetes (nearly invariably caused by excess weight and sedentary lifestyle)
- has high cholesterol
- has high blood pressure

Men with all four risk factors raise their risk of dementia nearly two and a half times over men with none of these risk factors. By the way, the sharper ones among you will have noticed that all the risk factors for dementia also apply to heart disease (see below). Award yourselves an extra point for that sharpness.

Other risk factors that have come out in other studies include:

- gum disease (probably because of the link with inflammation—see below)
- restricted social activity
- having an unchallenging job
- suffering higher levels of chronic stress

So what should you do? Of all the healthy lifestyle habits to adopt if you want to minimize your risk of dementia later on, perhaps the most important is exercise. It is abundantly clear that the more active you are in midlife, the lower your risk of dementia as you age.

How much exercise is needed? No one really knows, of course, but clearly at least the same amount of exercise that also limits the onslaught of heart disease and strokes and diabetes (see Chapter 7). And that's not really very much. For example, one study published in the *Journal of the American Medical Association* found that senior citizens who walked as little as two miles a day had half the risk of developing dementia as did seniors who were sedentary.

A good diet also never hurts and may even be of some help. For example, a recent study found that Japanese seniors who drank four or more glasses of fruit or vegetable juice a day had significantly lower risks of dementia than seniors who drank less juice. Anything magical in fruit or veggie juice? I doubt it. It's probably more that the juice intake was a marker for a better overall diet. After all, if you're into tomato juice instead of Coke with your meals, you're probably eating more nutritious foods, too. Other studies have linked specific dietary constituents (dark-skinned fruits, berries, green leafy veggies, whole grains) with better brain function in old age. So don't worry, eat berries.

Attitude also seems to matter. Thus, from the Religious Orders Study, researchers have concluded that those people who are most prone to "distress" in their thinking—that is, those who are most neurotic, believing that every situation is bound to turn out badly for them (well, doesn't it always?)—are also far more prone to Alzheimer's disease than are the most level-headed people. So don't worry, be happy.

As well, since smoking and drinking too much alcohol are also linked to higher risks of dementia, although not specifically to Alzheimer's disease, don't smoke or drink too much alcohol. A moderate intake of alcohol, however, might actually be protective against Alzheimer's disease and several other forms of dementia. So don't worry, drink happy.

Another key way to keep the brain more intact as we age is through "mental" exercise. Thus, a study from Columbia University found that people with fewer than eight years of school or those with less-skilled jobs (such as, I suppose, radio talk show hosts and men who work as city planners) had double the risk of Alzheimer's disease as those who had a more advanced education or higher-skilled jobs. This study also found that once Alzheimer's disease did set in, its course was not affected by level of education. In other words, it's probable that the more you use your brain in your younger years, the more synapses you develop, the larger the effective "usable" brain area you end up with, and the more capacity you have to draw on with the inevitable shrinkage and changes that the years will bring. So if you do nothing else, get yourself a good education, and you could clearly combine two benefits if you ran to your classes. If you don't already have an advanced degree, however, I doubt that buying one now from one of those mail-order universities will do the trick.

But don't get bummed out if you didn't get an advanced degree when you were younger. Studies also show that people who participate in activities that use their brain more (figuring out odds on horses, determining how many two-by-fours a project will require, determining how many beers the guys will need if the game goes into overtime) also lower their risk of dementia compared with guys who just go, "Yes, dear."

Of special note, many studies have linked the regular use of anti-inflammatory drugs, including ASA, to a lower risk of Alzheimer's disease. However, since scientists still do not know how these drugs work in the brain (is it an anti-inflammatory effect or is it something else?) or even if they really do work at all (is this simply a spurious association?), for now you would be best off not using these potent drugs regularly if the only reason you want to use them is to ward off dementia. The risks—bleeding, some kinds of strokes, ruptured ulcers—may be greater than the benefit.

As well, several studies have posed an intriguing link between the use of statin drugs (see below) and lowered risks of Alzheimer's disease. This, too, is something that needs lots more work, but the good news is that if you are already taking statins to lower your cholesterol levels, as so many of us are, you may be getting a double bang for your buck (actually a triple bang, since statin use has also been linked to lower rates of some cancers).

Among the proscriptions still commonly offered to minimize the risks of Alzheimer's disease is the one about avoiding aluminum, a potential toxin to the brain, although it's clearly much more likely that Alzheimer's is due to normal changes we all suffer as a result of aging and poor lifestyle habits than to the amount of aluminum-containing antacids we may swallow over our lifetimes.

Back Pain

The bad news is that 80 per cent of adults have experienced at least one episode of acute back pain by the time they hit fifty. The good news is that only about 10 per cent of us develop chronic back pain, so for most of us, acute back pain is a one-off or two-off or maybe even three-off event that responds equally well to any intervention we choose, mainly because the most important aspect of any treatment is what doctors call "tincture of time." (A trade secret, folks, so please don't tell anyone: tincture of time is the most important ingredient in nearly everything we prescribe. That will be thirty dollars, please.)

For those guys who simply cannot wait and who require—or more accurately, desire—more than a passing pat on the back when they're hurting and the "You're all right, dear" reassurance that all of our women friends are so quick to offer us when we're in indescribably severe pain, the best thing is to take a few mild analgesics or anti-inflammatories and try to return to normal activity as soon as possible. The drugs may or may not work (I doubt that they do very much for most of us), but as quick a return to normal activity as possible is vital. The longer you lie in bed feeling sorry for yourself, the poorer your prognosis. It's not the feeling sorry for yourself that's a concern (hey, all men need a bit of TLC—or a lot of it—when they're in pain), it's the bed rest. While lying around and doing nothing for weeks on end may give you something in common with your teenage son, it actually does your back lots of harm by allowing the pain to linger, since the muscles and other soft tissues, like your son, quickly get used to doing nothing and signal their resentment when even normal activities are reintroduced by sending out painful signals.

As to more active therapies, it's usually not necessary to get any of these, but if you want to go to someone, keep in mind that most studies conclude that it doesn't matter much which intervention you choose—chiropractic manipulation, physiotherapy, massage, eating cheese, even, according to a recent study, psychological counselling to help you "understand your pain" (What's there to understand? It hurts, dammit.)—because they all offer equally effective relief.

"I can buy getting back to work quickly, Art," I can hear some of you whining, "and I can even buy not getting any therapy for my sore back. But what I find hard to accept is that you haven't suggested getting any tests—X-rays or CT scans—to tell me that I don't have a ruptured disk that might paralyze me in an instant." Sorry, Jack, it's very rare that you will need such tests because very few cases of acute back pain require investigation. That doesn't mean that tests won't occasionally reveal a bulging disk. They often do because lots of us develop one or more bulging disks in our spinal column as we get older. The thing is, though, that these bulging disks are usually incidental to aging and seldom the cause of the back pain we're complaining of. If a surgeon sees one of those incidental bulging discs, however, he may be very tempted to go in and fix it. An old joke: One surgeon says to another, "What did the patient have?" "Eight hundred dollars." "No. I mean what did you operate for?" "I told you—eight hundred dollars."

Having said that, you should see your physician immediately if you develop:

- sudden sharp back pain that is accompanied by weakness (difficulty moving a part) in any of your lower limbs, especially your feet or ankles
- pain that is accompanied by any difficulty with urination or bowel movements
- pain that is severe and unrelenting, especially if it is getting worse
- sharp back pain that is accompanied by fever and chills (not chills from the natural fear all men have of even minor pain but chills as a sign of infection)

Finally, acute back pain is preventable if you follow some simple rules, most of which your mom told you:

- Keep your weight down (duh!) since back pain is directly related to excess weight.
- Don't smoke (smokers have way more back pain than nonsmokers).
- When you have to lift boxes or furniture—as when your wife decides to redesign the living room for the second time that week—bend properly and lift only from the knees. Better still, get your wife to do her own damn lifting.
- Maintain good posture: remember your mom's voice (I don't have to remember it; it's always on hand) and sit up straight. Straighter.
- Don't watch too much TV because studies show that when we watch TV or work at a computer for hours on end, we tend to slouch much more than when sitting in other situations, and we end up with much more back pain as a consequence.
- Most important, keep in shape, especially by doing "core" muscle exercises. And I can vouch for that one, folks, because since I started my exercise regimen with all those stupid crunches they make me do every two days, my incidence of back pain has sharply decreased.

As to the type of surface to sleep on, opinions differ about which mattress is best, but I figure it's not the type of mattress you sleep on as much as the type of partner you choose to sleep with that matters most.

One final note about preventing back pain: there's absolutely no proof—none at all—that all the manipulation in the world can prevent anyone's back from hurting from time to time. Regular manipulation sure prevents the chiropractor from going broke by having an empty office, though.

Colorectal Cancer

Breast cancer affects one in nine North American women, a "factoid" that most of you undoubtedly can recite when called on because breast cancer organizations have been very successful at selling that particular statistic to the public (although like all bare statistics, this one also needs a lot of interpretation—that will come in my next book, of course). And because you read the chapter on prostate cancer so carefully, you can also cite the fact, I'm sure, that roughly one in six men will end up with prostate cancer.

But I'm willing to bet my Bob Dylan vinyl albums against your Rolling Stones vinyl albums (I always had better taste) that most of you don't have even an inkling that roughly one in fourteen North Americans end up with colorectal cancer. And I'm also willing to bet my Calvins against your Polos (see what I said earlier?) that most of you don't know colorectal cancer hits both genders equally hard, making it currently the second leading cause of cancer death in North America (after another equal-opportunity malignancy, lung cancer), a fact that is very frustrating to everyone in the medical business because so many deaths from colorectal cancer are preventable. Most colon cancers start in the lining of the bowel as precancerous changes known as adenomatous polyps, which are relatively easy to detect (see below) and remove at their benign, premalignant stage.

So let's get down to it, guys: who gets colorectal cancer and why do they get it? Some of the key risk factors for colorectal cancer include:

- age: as always, the older you are, the higher your risk
- family history
- genetic profile: Ashkenazi Jews, for example, such as your author, are especially prone to colon cancer (more ammunition to make my mom feel guilty—never works, though), as are people of Chinese descent
- a history of adenomatous polyps
- a history of one of several bowel-related conditions, including ulcerative colitis, hereditary nonpolyposis colorectal cancer, and familial adenomatous polyposis

Clearly there's not a whole lot you can do about the aforementioned risk factors (you don't, for example, want to stop growing older because the alternative has several major disadvantages, not the least being the current cost of burials, although that's probably more of a concern to your offspring than it is to you), but happily, as always, there are several lifestyle risk factors for colorectal cancer that you can do something about. The non-controversial ones include:

- smoking
- obesity
- heavy alcohol use
- not doing exercise

The controversial lifestyle factor linked to an increased risk of colorectal cancer is diet. Thus, it's commonly claimed that you will protect yourself against colon cancer, if you eat more:

- fibre
- fruit and veggies
- antioxidant- and vitamin-rich foods
- calcium
- whole grains
- folate-containing foods

And it's claimed that you will raise your risk of colon cancer if you eat a diet high in:

- meat, especially red meat
- saturated fat and trans fat
- protein
- high glycemic index foods
- calories

The problem is that studies attempting to show that appropriate dietary changes (such as eating more fibre or taking more vitamins) can help people who've been diagnosed with precancerous polyps don't indicate that people end up reducing their eventual risk of colon cancer.

But as a firm believer in the benefits of a healthy diet for all your body parts, not just your bowel, my response to such inconclusive studies is that they've been looking at the wrong end—of your life, that is. What I mean is that by the time your end ends up with polyps, it's probably too late to hope that dietary changes will make much difference to your cancer risk.

If, however, you start on a good diet earlier in your life, like, say, with your next meal, then I am certain a healthy Mediterranean diet (see Chapter 6) will very likely reduce your risk of several types of malignancy, including colorectal cancer.

Interestingly, several studies have also linked the regular use of both ASA and statin drugs with a lower risk of colorectal cancer, although it's far too soon to advise taking either ASA or statins simply in order to help your back end. If, however, you're already taking ASA or a statin to improve your heart disease risks, then hey, you're sitting on good news, friend.

Signs and symptoms of colorectal cancer include:

- ongoing feelings of bloating or cramping or pain in the abdomen
- a persistent change in bowel habits, especially the development of constipation and/or narrower stools (As an intern, I once made the mistake of asking an elderly veteran of both world wars if he had developed ribbon-like stools, and his response made it instantly clear that it was a damn good thing I'd never had to serve under his command. So, be forewarned: Canadian vets don't pay much attention to their stools, and if they do, they certainly don't want to talk about it with you.)
- a feeling that you still (in the words of that famous bowel specialist, my wife) "have to poo" after you've had a bowel movement
- blood in your stool or bleeding from the rectum

So I guess this is as good a time as any to advise you that, so long as you don't serve in the Canadian army, you must develop the habit of examining your after-effects regularly, and if you're one of those anal-retentive goyim who've never learned to look behind yourself and you want a quick sure-fire strategy to overcome your embarrassment about seeing what's there, just spend some time with a Jewish mother. It'll cure you, right quick.

That said, I also know that many men who read this book and who've learned to swear by all the other great advice they've garnered herein will take this latest admonishment to heart, too, and will undoubtedly develop the habit of avidly examining every one of their stools for signs of malignancy, and some will consequently start to worry excessively about every tiny speck of blood they find on the toilet paper, or every too-thin bowel movement they deposit. So before you become too frightened and consequently too reckless with this strategy, let me warn you of the potential drawbacks.

First, you can seriously strain your neck from too many too careful examinations of this sort. Second, spending too much time in such activities can detract from more important jobs, such as relating to your family in the morning ("Is Dad locking himself in the bathroom again, Mom?"), and besides, what if you forget to lock the door and your fifteen-year-old walks in and catches you on your hands and knees? Believe me, you won't ever earn enough to pay for her therapy. But most important, you shouldn't get too nervous about the foregoing (or should that really be "aftergoing") because the majority of people with such symptoms have nothing seriously wrong with them. If the symptoms are persistent, however, get them checked out.

As stated earlier, most colorectal cancers start as precancerous polyps, and the average polyp takes about ten years to turn into a malignancy. Happily, polyps are very easy to remove surgically, thus preventing them from turning into cancers.

You have to find them first, though. So starting sometime in midlife (your fears, your other needs, and your risk profiles will help determine a good age at which to start), you should begin to get regular rectal examinations, yes, from a doctor, and yes, it's done exactly the same and with the same number of digits as is the dreaded DRE for prostate cancer (see Chapter 4).

But that's only a start because a rectal exam really only covers the territory that a digit can cover, and that's not very far, especially if your doctor is someone like me with very small hands and very small fingers.

It's even more important, starting in midlife, to get more sophisticated screening tests for colorectal cancer. Certainly, the most common, most easily done, and most available screening test is a stool test for occult blood. In the most common version of a stool test for occult blood, the patient collects three samples of stool and submits them (on a special card, to be sure, and with a degree of delicacy) to the lab, where they are checked for microscopic amounts of blood, which is shed by polyps and cancers (and other benign lesions, too). If the stool test is positive, that person is subjected to more exact testing (see below).

Now what could be easier than that? I ask. I mean, even people who work for the Department of Fisheries can remember that sequence, I'm sure, although some of them may not be able to count up to three too reliably, but hey, they can at least do it once. And the benefits of a stool test for occult blood are obvious. This test is:

- easy to complete
- portable (although I do think it's better done at home, and I mean your own home)
- reliable (several studies have shown that annual screening with stool tests for occult blood can save lots of lives)

- private (not necessarily if you happen to live with a teenager)
- very cheap (its best feature for the bureaucrats who have to pay for such things)

Despite these advantages, studies show that a stool test for occult blood is a test generally honoured in the breach. Why? Simply because most of you hate doing it. There's just something about smearing your, well, you know what, on a card and sharing that card with a stranger that doesn't seem to ring a lot of bells for most of you (although, I'd bet more of you would be willing to do it if you could send the card to, say, your city hall than to your doctor's office). But guys, you can't do that (or at least you shouldn't, in large part because your mayor isn't qualified to read it), so since this is a very important test that might just save your life, I'd advise you instead to do it the right way. This involves sitting yourself down in the throne room with a good read (such as this book, but others will work equally well); doing what you have to do, or even if you don't have to do it, doing it anyway; and when you're ready, taking a deep breath (it helps to breathe ahead of time, and don't forget to put the book down first); and then, as in those Swoosh ads, just doing it, three times in a row (well, the sooner it's done, the better for everyone sharing that room, right?). And yes, you have to repeat it every year, but it gets easier with practice. Well, no, it doesn't, but it doesn't get harder, either.

While stool tests for occult blood are effective screening tools for a large population, for the individual, the best and most effective screening tools for colon cancer are either routine sigmoidoscopy or colonoscopy (although some doctors still recommend barium X-rays for some patients). For both of these procedures, you get to lie on a table in a very undignified manner (knees up, Doctor Hister) while a doctor first does a digital rectal exam on you (Hey! Who's gonna argue in that position, and besides, do you really want to antagonize the doctor at that particular moment?), and then shoves a flexible tube (that's how doctors describe that rigid band of steel, at any rate) up where the sun will never shine. A gastroenterologist friend of mine who does a lot of these procedures describes them as "a case of one arsehole looking up another arsehole," and you know, it's not for me to say this, but he's right.

In a sigmoidoscopy, the tube goes only (I use the word simply in a comparative sense, of course) part way through the large bowel, although in the end, it has to go up there pretty far, and unfortunately, studies have indicated that some doctors who do sigmoidoscopies just don't go up far enough, so that patients screened with sigmoidoscopies, particularly elderly individuals, can end up with a pretty large number of colorectal cancers that might have been detected with more thorough procedures. Bottom line: if this is the way you choose to be screened, push your doctor to push his way in as far as he can go.

Going only part way through the bowel is not at all a problem with a colonoscopy because the doctor goes for the Whopper right from the get-go, shoving the tip end of the scope all the way into the right side of the colon (and sometimes beyond; the major complication of colonoscopies is bowel perforation). So of all the screening tests, colonoscopies have the best rate of colon cancer detection, although they are the most labour-intensive and most costly. Been there, by the way, and had it done (three times, in fact), and all I can say is that I never felt a thing, mostly because I was completely out while it was being done, although according to my gastroenterologist I was only "lightly sedated." (I'm sure he didn't want me asking questions while he was enjoying his work: "So what's for lunch later, Lawrie?") That said, I must tell you that by far the worst part of this procedure for me was the prep, which involved drinking a gallon of what tasted exactly like a soapy salty solution (which it was, of course) the night before and feeling wretched the entire night and following day. Next time, I lie about how much of the solution I've taken.

More recently, the idea of "virtual" colonoscopies has grabbed a lot of headlines, but before you leap to the conclusion that this will surely be much more tolerable since it involves a computer-generated image of your insides, thus obviating the need, you figure, to be prepped, let me instantly explode that notion for you. Virtual colonoscopy, or computed tomographic colonography, does indeed involve the use of computer-generated images of the insides of the bowel, and it has the added advantage that it can see surrounding areas as well. But you still need to be cleaned out properly to get it done, so it's still prep school for you, I'm afraid.

How often should you get these screening tests and which ones should you get? That all depends on your risk profile (some of us need to be screened more often than others do, and hey! I hate you for that), and your and your doctor's preferences.

Diabetes

Diabetes affects 6 to 7 per cent of the population (although about half of all diabetics don't know they have the disease—see below), an increase of 41 per cent since 1997, and this percentage is expected to rise dramatically over the next thirty years, not only because diabetes is now being diagnosed in baby boomers in much higher numbers and often up to two decades earlier than in our parents, but also because it's begun to be diagnosed in our overly fat kids at alarmingly early ages. This is especially true, alas, in some genetic groups (including aboriginal peoples and South Asians) that seem to be at particularly high risk for this disorder. Thus, researchers tell us that although Type II diabetes was never seen in Canada's native population fifty years ago, it is now being diagnosed in that population at over three times the rate that is seen in non-natives.

Diabetes is a complex metabolic disorder in which an abnormally high blood glucose (sugar) level damages both large and small arteries and the tissues those arteries service. There are two types of diabetes, cunningly named Type I diabetes and Type II diabetes. In Type I diabetes, which accounts for 10 per cent of all cases, pancreas cells are destroyed, nearly always early in life—hence the old name of juvenile-onset diabetes—resulting in an eventual disappearance of insulin in the bloodstream. Thus, Type I diabetics require lifelong insulin replacement, unless, that is, researchers come up with a successful pancreatic tissue transplant that is able to secrete insulin in its new transplanted home. The great news is that they're getting much closer to finding an effective way to transplant pancreas cells and keep them alive and functioning. The bad news is that they still have a long way to go.

Type II diabetes accounts for about 90 per cent of all diabetes cases, and is largely the offspring of an inappropriate lifestyle that eventually causes the body to become "resistant" to its own insulin. What that means is that in Type II diabetes, the patient starts with enough insulin to do what insulin is supposed to do, then for reasons that are still not fully understood, but that clearly involve carrying excess weight and living a sedentary lifestyle, the body becomes unable to respond normally to its own insulin. The pancreas tries to do its part by producing more and more of that ineffective insulin, and eventually, if Type II diabetes lasts long enough, the pancreas runs out of insulin.

The most prevalent theory about why we are witnessing an epidemic of Type II diabetes is that human beings have simply outstripped evolution (although even its proponents admit that this theory flies in the face of such strong empirical counterevidence as Donald Trump, Cher, curling, Trailer Park Boys, and infomercials). This theory postulates that our ancestors lived in a constant feast-or-famine state. When they managed to down a mastodon or a sabre-toothed tiger, they gorged on the carcass (at least our carnivore ancestors did; the ones who preferred veggies or tofu probably never made it up the evolutionary ladder), and their bodies learned to burn the calories quickly and store what wasn't needed right away as fat, since they could not predict when the next feast or even the next meal would be served up. We, however, are privileged to feast every day, and in the case of my sons several times a day, and our metabolic processes have simply not kept up. Thus, although we don't need all the extra fat those supplemental calories give us, we store the fat anyway, leading to the metabolic changes of Type II diabetes.

It's important to note, though, that diabetes is just the end stage of a continuum of abnormal glucose and insulin metabolism and that long before you get diagnosed formally with diabetes, you are still suffering the consequences of insulin resistance. This condition—increasing insulin resistance without any change yet in glucose levels—has had several names, including prediabetes, and is now known as a key component of the metabolic syndrome.

The metabolic syndrome has itself gone through more redefinitions than Michael Jackson, but the most recent definition from the International Diabetes Federation is this: for a person to be diagnosed with the metabolic syndrome, they must have "central" obesity (also known as abdominal obesity) as well as at least two of the following four characteristics:

- reduced HDL (see below)
- high triglycerides (ditto)
- high blood pressure
- raised glucose levels (the result, nearly invariably, of insulin resistance)

Some experts also want to add other factors such as raised levels of inflammatory proteins and clotting factors, but for now, we'll stick with these five.

Want an even easier way to tell who's got the metabolic syndrome without resorting to blood tests? Just look around you (or more frightening, just look down) and anyone with a dome for a profile very likely has the metabolic syndrome.

Why is this syndrome so important? Because studies show that even in a prediabetic state, you are already suffering damage to your arteries, leading to higher risks of heart attack, strokes, blindness, dementia, and of course, the most dreaded consequence of all, sudden premature death.

Risk factors for Type II diabetes include:

- being overweight
- following a calorie-rich diet with an overabundance of refined carbohydrates and trans fats in it

- getting older
- living a sedentary life
- having had a previous blood test showing impaired glucose tolerance
- having a parent with Type II diabetes

Weight gain and sedentary lifestyle, though, stand out as chief risk factors. In fact, some experts now refer to the rise in diabetes cases that are associated with obesity as the "diabesity" epidemic. Thus, nine of ten newly diagnosed American diabetics in 2003 were overweight. Further, several studies have shown that even very modest weight loss—five to ten pounds—can lower the risk of developing Type II diabetes, and can even help a newly diagnosed diabetic avoid having to take drugs. As well, any exercise at all has been found to be preventive against Type II diabetes. And the beneficial effect of exercise on glucose levels and insulin levels can go on for several weeks after the exercise is over.

Clearly, not everyone is at equal risk of developing Type II diabetes from weight gain alone. After all, we all know some very thin people who became diabetic while we also know some very heavy folks who never develop diabetes. Both, I'm afraid, are prisoners of their genes, so while the former were genetically condemned to illness despite their best attempts to avoid it, the latter are happy simpletons who are genetically protected no matter what they do, probably because God didn't want to punish them more than She already had. You and I, Jocko, are usually not that lucky, however, and God is quite happy to punish us for even our minor transgressions, and diabetes seems to be one of Her preferred ways.

Why is diabetes such a big deal? Because diabetics have higher rates of:

- stroke
- heart attack: 75 to 80 per cent of diabetics will die of a cardiovascular complication, and yet, studies show, most diabetics are not aware of the link between heart disease and diabetes; also of note is the fact that since diabetes leads to nerve damage (see below), diabetics might not even be able to feel the early signs of angina warning them of impending cardiac trouble
- erectile dysfunction: this is practically a one to one relationship—that is, if you have diabetes, you will also end up with ED, but only if you're a male, of course
- blindness
- amputation (especially of the lower limbs)
- kidney failure

- nerve damage: signs of nerve damage, such as pain from even the light touch of a sock or loss of sensation so that even very painful sensations are not felt, will develop in nearly half those people who have Type II diabetes within ten years of being diagnosed, yet one study found that only 10 per cent of diabetics knew about this very disturbing complication
- painful and often intractable skin ulcers
- dementia: diabetics are up to three times more likely to suffer from dementia than their nondiabetic brothers
- some types of cancer, most notably of the colon
- depression: one huge survey found that diabetics are twice as likely as non-diabetics to suffer from both depression and chronic anxiety

Do I have to *emphasize* this for you? Well, maybe I will, just in case. *This is a disease very much worth preventing.*

It's easy to diagnose Type II diabetes in someone who starts drinking huge amounts of water, who runs to the bathroom several extra times a day (and night), who is very hungry, and who is also feeling very tired and losing weight. But 50 per cent of people with Type II diabetes don't know they have it (the average diabetic is said to have diabetes for six years before it is diagnosed), because in the early stages the symptoms are either nonexistent or very subtle.

So watching for symptoms is not an adequate way to tell if you need to be concerned about your blood sugar levels. Instead, it just makes sense for middle-aged men to have blood glucose tests (and other tests for the metabolic syndrome—see Chapter 1) on a regular basis. According to the Canadian Task Force on Preventive Health Care, "impaired fasting glucose is diagnosed if the fasting glucose level is 6.1 to 6.9 mmol/L," while the American Diabetes Association claims that 100 to 125 mg/dL indicates impaired fasting levels.

If you have already developed Type II diabetes, to control your blood sugar levels you must:

- Get down as close to your desirable weight as you can (and I don't mean the weight you desire to get to, which is probably thirty pounds too much, but the weight the charts tell you is the most desirable for your height).
- Start doing exercise (as little exercise as a brisk daily two- or three-mile walk of thirty to forty minutes is enough to help most people control blood sugar levels, but the more you do, the better control you will achieve, and the lower your risk of premature death—something we all want to aim for).
- Moderate your consumption of alcohol (although moderate alcohol intake

protects against developing diabetes, excess alcohol intake can play havoc with blood sugar levels).

- Limit your intake of high-calorie, high-fat foods, and refined carbohydrates, and increase your intake of antioxidant-rich fruits and vegetables, as well as legumes and whole grains.

You may also want to try taking chromium supplements. The jury is still out on how beneficial these can be for diabetics, but several studies have indicated that supplemental chromium may lower the risk of cardiac complications in Type II diabetes. Do this only with full knowledge of your doctor, though.

Nearly all Type II diabetics should also take prophylactic ASA (see below), and nearly all should be taking a statin drug to lower their cholesterol levels, even if those cholesterol levels are "normal" (see below) because diabetics need much lower LDL levels than nondiabetics do, so while an LDL of up to 3.2 mmol/L may be OK for a low-risk nondiabetic, diabetics should aim for 2.5 and below, if possible.

Diabetics must also aim for blood pressures that are lower than those set for nondiabetics (see below). These things are always changing but for now, a diabetic should aim for a blood pressure below 130/80.

And again, the lower the better, as long as the blood pressure does not lead to symptoms. It's also very important to have frequent blood tests to help you gauge how well you are controlling your blood sugar levels. I don't mean just those blood glucose tests you can do on your own at home—you must also have the more specialized HbA1c test that monitors how well you're controlling your blood sugar over the long term.

Several medications help control blood sugar, and researchers are also actively pursuing revolutionary new therapies such as transplantation of pancreatic cells, insulin in pill form, and artificial pancreases.

Unfortunately, far too many diabetics are not doing enough to control their illness. And too many doctors are not offering diabetics the medications—ASA, statins—that might prolong their lives. In fact, a recent American study concluded that "diabetes is out of control" with two out of three Type II diabetics not controlling their blood sugar levels nearly well enough, which is very worrisome when added to other studies that show most people being treated for high blood pressure never get their blood pressure down to a normal range, and that most people with high cholesterol levels do not achieve target goals for cholesterol. Sadly, this does not bode well for the future.

Gastroesophageal Reflux Disease

In gastroesophageal reflux disease (GERD), hydrochloric acid washes back from the stomach into the esophagus. Now as you would expect, the esophagus is no different from you and me. It doesn't enjoy getting burned by acid, and eventually the washed-up acid irritates the esophagus enough to produce esophagitis, or inflammation of the esophagus. Most people with esophageal reflux are able to control it with appropriate therapy, but in about a quarter of cases esophagitis becomes recurrent, persistent, and progressive, and eventually the irritated and altered esophageal lining can develop premalignant changes. Chew on that news for a while as you swallow another antacid, or three.

A quick aside about hiatus hernia, which is often confused with reflux. A hiatus hernia occurs when the diaphragm weakens. The diaphragm is the muscle that separates the thoracic cavity, which contains the lungs and heart, from the abdominal cavity, which contains the stomach and bowels and other bits. There is a tight opening in the diaphragm through which the esophagus slides into the stomach, and when that tight opening widens, parts of the stomach can slide upwards, creating a hiatus hernia. A hiatus hernia can be silent, and it can also be associated with reflux, but just because you are diagnosed with a hiatus hernia does not necessarily mean you have reflux disease too. And vice versa.

Gastroesophageal reflux is extremely common. Thirty per cent of adults experience symptoms frequently, and 10 per cent of us have daily symptoms.

Reflux has been associated with many risk factors, including:

- smoking
- obesity
- snoring
- eating large, fatty meals
- insomnia
- excess alcohol intake
- ingesting coffee and caffeinated products
- being sedentary
- having asthma (see below)
- eating lots of salt
- high blood pressure
- the use of sleeping pills
- the use of other drugs such as alendronate (Fosamax) for osteoporosis
- drinking carbonated beverages in the late afternoon or evening

The symptoms most commonly associated with reflux are:

- regurgitation of stomach contents into the mouth
- indigestion
- heartburn, which is really any burning sensation from just north of the belly button to the back of the throat
- abdominal pain

Reflux disease can also rear its ugly head by producing:

- chest pain
- hoarseness, especially in the morning (after you have been lying down for several hours and the acid has had a field night inflaming your throat)
- a persistent sore throat
- and the symptom that I particularly want to flag—coughing or wheezing, especially at night

This last, nocturnal asthma, is often caused or aggravated by the washing up of acid to irritate the airways when you lie down, and asthmatics who wake up wheezing and hacking and feeling short of breath, despite seemingly adequate treatment of their asthma, should consider their stomachs a possible source of their persistent symptoms.

Gastroesophageal reflux disease is most accurately diagnosed not by an expert or a celebrity you saw on *Oprah* who discussed how his life had radically changed the day he accepted GERD into his life but by investigations that involve a look down the gullet and into the stomach. If this kind of validation were required for every case, however, gastroenterologists would be so busy looking down the bow that they would have no time left for the stern, an end many of these guys actually prefer for reasons I refuse to speculate about. Thus, most suspected cases of gastroesophageal reflux disease in middle age can and should be treated first with a trial of therapy, and only when this fails or when the condition is persistent or progressive should further investigation be undertaken.

To improve reflux, you should take the following steps:

- Lose some weight because the more you weigh, the worse your symptoms.
- Wait several hours after a meal before lying down.
- Avoid straining (even bending over) and exercising after eating.
- Do not wear a tight belt (or if you do, wear it plumber-fashion down around your knees; you may get the pulchritude police after you, but at least you won't be burping and belching when they show up).

- Don't smoke.
- Do some exercise. In one study, as little as 30 minutes of exercise once a week was enough to cut the rate of GERD by 50 per cent.
- Chew gum. Chewing gum stimulates saliva production and this seems to help neutralize acid in the esophagus.
- Elevate the head of your bed. Some experts advise putting phone books under the head of the bed, although if your reflux is as persistent as mine, you probably won't get relief from postural drainage even if you sleep standing up.
- Sleep more on your left side.
- Avoid any trigger you recognize that worsens your symptoms (duh!).

As to dietary changes, it's the usual whole enchilada. Actually, an enchilada might not be a good idea, since fatty foods put a strain on the esophageal-stomach barrier and make reflux worse. Go easy on alcohol and caffeine, although in a recent survey, a majority of people with reflux claimed that coffee did not make their symptoms worse (you gotta admire just how much self-delusion coffee lovers will go through in order to keep drinking their favourite brew), and avoid foods that may worsen symptoms, such as:

- chocolate (Doesn't bother me. Self-delusion? Moi?)
- vinegar products
- onions
- bananas (a particular bane for my reflux)
- carbonated drinks
- citrus fruits and juices
- peppermint
- tomato products

Also, don't eat within at least three hours of going to bed, and try to eat small, less fatty, more frequent meals rather than one or two large ones.

Most people with gastroesophageal reflux disease self-medicate with antacids or acid-suppressing drugs, and these drugs certainly work well in mild cases, but you should never self-medicate for more than a few weeks without discussing your persistent symptoms with a physician. When you have to move beyond self-medication, and most of you will have to, there are a host of drugs to choose from. The most popular and most effective are proton pump inhibitors (PPIs) such as omeprazole, which work very well, although be warned that a potential side effect, according to a recent study, is a significantly increased risk of developing pneumonia (probably because PPIs do such a good job suppressing stomach acid, and stomach acid may be an important defence against the pathogens that cause pneumonia), and that the complete safety of PPIs over the long term has not been completely established, although they have been around for thirty years and the data so far are very reassuring. One other key problem with these drugs is a significant rebound increase in acid output when you try to come off them, something I've discovered to my chagrin each time I've tried to discontinue them. You are not me, though, and you should manage to come off these drugs if you are persistent and if you slowly taper your dose.

Remember also that if you have to take any of these drugs for chronic persistent esophagitis, you may need to have your esophagus looked into from time to time to make sure that you're not developing early precancerous changes of the esophagus.

When the drugs don't work, or when people tire of taking a constant run of drugs, many turn to surgery, which involves tightening the muscle that separates the stomach from the esophagus. Several different procedures have been developed for this condition but the principle is the same: it's harder for acid to run back though a tighter sphincter.

Be aware, however, that the long-term results of this surgery have not been stellar, so that according to several followups, most people who've had the surgery still require the use of some medication to keep their reflux in check.

Heart Disease

To understand heart disease, the number one killer in North America, you need to know about arteries. Atherosclerotic disease refers to the narrowing of arteries due to the buildup of fatty substances, calcium, inflammatory cells, clotting material, and other products in plaques on the inside of any artery wall. This comes about when toxic factors such as cigarette smoke and oxidized LDL cholesterol (and perhaps inflammatory proteins resulting from gum disease or even the flu) damage the lining of the blood vessels, which prompts the body to bring in the troops (white cells, anti-inflammatory cells, anti-clotting proteins, and so on) to allay the inflammation. The paradox here is that all the gunk (that's a very technical term) that arrives at the site of blood vessel inflammation, both the helpful stuff and the damaging stuff, contributes to the further buildup of the plaques on the insides of the vessel walls. When this occurs in the arteries that supply blood to the heart, it constitutes coronary heart disease (CHD). Most heart attacks occur because unstable coronary plaques split or rupture, provoking an even more intense protective reaction in that area of the blood vessel, which in turn significantly raises the risk of a blood clot forming that plugs the artery completely. This prevents blood from reaching the parts of the heart tissue supplied by that now plugged artery and is called a heart attack.

Symptoms

The classic symptoms of a heart attack include:

- chest pain that is usually described as crushing or vicelike and that can radiate to the jaw, neck, left arm, or back
- sweating
- anxiety
- nausea
- shortness of breath, also known as SOB (curiously, SOB also often describes the guy who's just had a heart attack, and many times his doctor as well)

That's the classic picture. We now know, however, that substantial numbers of people have "atypical" heart attack symptoms that include:

- right-sided chest pain
- throat discomfort
- chest discomfort and aches rather than crushing pain
- pressure on the chest
- weakness
- vomiting
- indigestion

As well, many people complain of symptoms that precede their heart attack, sometimes for days and weeks, including unusual fatigue, shortness of breath, indigestion, and intense anxiety.

The reason it's important to make note of both the acute symptoms and those that are harbingers of a heart attack is that lots of people don't recognize these symptoms for what they are: an impending cardiac crisis. Thus, they often do little to prevent the heart problem from worsening, and even worse, they don't get to hospital fast enough after they've suffered the heart attack. When it comes to treating a heart attack, time is incredibly important because in this era of clot-busting medications, the faster you get to treatment, the less permanent the damage you may suffer. So if you think you're suffering a heart attack, don't phone your wife to ask for advice or a lift to the ER. Swallow an ASA tablet as fast as you can, call 9-1-1, and get to the hospital. ASAP. (Full disclosure forces me to admit that the day I had crushing chest pain, I drove around for hours waiting for it to disappear because I was certain that it was only esophageal spasm. Thank God, I was right. But boy, did I ever get some lectures in the ER when I finally showed up there.)

Also, I hesitate to say this, but doctors aren't always as correct in their diagnosis of heart attack as we can or should be. Thus, one study found that 3 per cent of three thousand people who'd visited emergency rooms with chest pain and who were told that their pain was not from their coronary arteries went on to suffer a full-fledged heart attack within the subsequent month. This was particularly true for people with high cholesterol and diabetes. So if you have symptoms that make you wary about your heart, be insistent that the doctors do all the tests they can do to help them with this diagnosis. It's your life, after all, not theirs that is at risk here.

Risk Factors

Factors related to a higher risk of heart disease include:

- advancing age
- a strong family history of premature heart disease or stroke
- abnormal cholesterol levels (high LDL and triglyceride levels, low HDL—see below)
- high blood pressure
- metabolic syndrome and diabetes
- central or abdominal obesity
- smoking
- being sedentary
- eating too few fruits and veggies
- experiencing excess stress
- abstaining from alcohol (although clearly there is a lot of debate about this one)

How important are these factors? Vital. In fact, according to a much-publicized Canadian study, that preceding list of risk factors accounts for 90 per cent of all heart attacks.

So let's take a closer look at some of those risks, beginning with the two you can't do much about, age and family history.

The older you are, the higher your risk, but you can't, or rather you shouldn't, do much to affect this risk factor.

Family history is similar. One middle-aged friend I know is a poster boy for the benefits of running, a health fiend who eats as nutritious a diet as can be eaten, and who has never smoked or done anything else to prematurely injure his blood vessels. Yet, one day, while on one of his regular long runs, he developed chest pain and was quickly found to have four very plugged cardiac arteries, which required a quadruple bypass procedure. When we talked about his illness subsequently, he shrugged and said, "I guess you can't outrun your genes." You see, his father and his brother had both suffered heart attacks at a young age.

He's right, of course. Your genes and your family history have a very significant influence on your risk of heart attack, so that if you have a male first-degree relative (father, brother) who had a heart attack before the age of fifty-five or a female first-degree relative who suffered a coronary event before the age of sixty-five, you have a much higher risk of suffering a heart attack yourself even if, as in my friend's example, you do all the right things to try to prevent a heart attack, and even if you have no evident symptoms of heart disease.

So if you have that ghost in your family, be particularly vigilant about the other risk factors that you can do something about.

Cholesterol Levels

To start, as always, some definitions. Lipids are fats (my kids, who clearly got their senses of humour from the wrong parent, have nicknamed me Lipid, by the way). Lipoproteins are compounds of fatty substances and proteins that serve as a transport system to deliver fats to your tissues. Most cholesterol, a type of fat, is carried in the bloodstream as part of low density lipoproteins (LDL), the so-called bad cholesterol. When LDL is oxidized and deposited into the walls of already damaged arteries, it injures those arteries even further (hence the benefits of a diet full of antioxidants). Some cholesterol is also carried as high density lipoproteins (HDL), the so-called good cholesterol, which gets its secondary moniker because HDL protects your arteries and inhibits some of the damage LDL can do. Triglycerides, high levels of which have also been linked to damage in coronary arteries, are fats carried in the blood on the backs of very low density lipoproteins (VLDL).

Now I realize that what you have just read is a real plateful, so if you're getting overwhelmed, all you have to remember is this: High HDL = Good.

High LDL = Bad. High VLDL = Bad. You got that? Good boy. So anything that helps raise your HDL levels is good for you, while anything that raises LDL levels consistently (trans fats, some saturated fats) can be bad for you because the more those LDL and VLDL transports steam into your already injured arteries to deposit their thick sludge and inflame those narrowed channels even more, the higher your risk of heart attack. Want a word picture? Just think of those cruise ships that visit Skagway or Vera Cruz and unload their tons of tubby tourists, who immediately inflame the natives and plug up the narrowed streets of the town they take over.

That said, as with love and a car rental charge, there is more to these fats equations than meets the eye because some people are genetically protected against damaging their arteries unduly no matter how little they do to protect themselves. These guys are the exceptions, however.

To ascertain your risk from the lipid convoy steaming into your coronary arteries, you need a full blood cholesterol profile, consisting of your total cholesterol level, LDL level, HDL level, triglyceride level, and VLDL level. Note that in Canada chlesterol levels are given in millimoles per litre (mmol/L) and in the U.S. levels are given in milligrams per decilitre (mg/dL).

Although the numbers vary a bit according to the organization promoting heart health, the Heart and Stroke Foundation of Canada gives these values for "good target levels":

- Total cholesterol: below 5.2 mmol/L (200 mg/dL)
- LDL: below 3.5 mmol/L (130 mg/dL), but you should aim lower
- HDL: above 1.0 mmol/L (40 mg/dL)

A word of warning, though. Focussing on your total cholesterol level only and ignoring the other numbers, as so many men and their doctors do, is akin to trying to figure out what a play is about by paying attention to only one character. If you are going to get your cholesterol levels checked, as I think every one of you should do at least once by middle age (and to hell with what the number-crunching health authorities and insurance companies think about the cost; if they're so keen to save tax and health care dollars, why don't they work for free? Fat chance, eh?), always get a full cholesterol profile. And then, be sure to remember the numbers.

You must also bear in mind that these are only general guidelines and that other risk factors must be considered along with cholesterol levels in evaluating the risk from those levels. Or to quote the wise words of an old free clinic hippie patient of mine whose name was Doc (I don't think he was an MD, although he was certainly a specialist in smoking), "Hey, dude! One man's high is just another man's mellow." Thus, it is now well established that a man with a family history of premature death from heart disease, for example, or one who has diabetes, requires intervention at lower LDL levels than does a man whose grandparents lived to a ripe old age and whose parents both expired in their nineties while making love for the third time that day. The latter guy may require some sort of different therapy, though.

Happily, most people who are told they have high cholesterol do not need to start on drugs immediately. Most can take a few months or longer to change their lifestyles to see how those changes affect their levels, and most of us can improve our cholesterol levels (and our heart attack risks) through appropriate lifestyle changes. Diet is always the number one risk factor to attack immediately, and the good news is that changes in diet can improve cholesterol levels by up to 30 per cent.

That said, changing your diet is not as straightforward as it used to seem because as studies on the Atkins diet have revealed, eating a lot more saturated fat doesn't necessarily lead to those worse cholesterol levels all the experts had promised such a diet would deliver. In fact, many people on high-protein, high-fat diets seem to benefit from improved cholesterol profiles, at least in the short term. Thus, the jury is out again on the best nutritional plan to follow if you want to improve your cholesterol levels, although if you ask me (and you bought this book, after all, so you must want to hear what I have to say) I would advise following one of two diets.

My favourite, because I find it both nutritious and delicious (equally important, of course) is a Mediterranean diet (see Chapter 6), which involves:

- eating way more fruits, veggies, grains, beans, and fibre
- eliminating as much trans fat from the diet as possible, lowering the intake of saturated fats, and instead focussing on monounsaturated fats such as olive oil
- decreasing your intake of meat, especially red meat
- increasing your intake of fish
- drinking a bit of wine regularly

Fairness in reporting, though, obliges me to tell you that the other diet that seems to work even better at improving LDL levels than a Mediterranean diet is what's come to be known as the Portfolio diet, which was put together by Dr. David Jenkins from the University of Toronto. The portfolio diet involves:

- increasing your intake of fruits and veggies
- substituting soy-based foods (soy burgers, breast of tofu, etc.) for meat
- eating lots of "sticky" fibre such as psyllium (yummy Metamucil), oats, eggplant, and okra
- using sterol-enriched margarine instead of butter or margarine
- eating lots of nuts, especially almonds

Now I have to tell you that Dr. Jenkins is a lovely and persuasive guy, who claims that eventually most people end up enjoying the Portfolio diet (although I have never quizzed him about how long that "eventually" ends up being), and every time I speak to him I come away certain that my intake of eggplant and okra is going to skyrocket that week since it's clear that full-scale adherence to the Portfolio diet results in LDL changes equivalent to the best results we get from cholesterol-lowering drugs. But try as I might, I'm just not an eggplant and okra and Metamucil kind of guy (I don't seem to have any problem with the almonds, though), and so I have not made much headway with the Portfolio diet. I fear that would be true for most of you, too, although if you can get around to eating this way, it's probably the healthiest diet you could follow. And remember, as Dr. Jenkins always stresses, you don't have to go whole hog for the Portfolio diet (although if you did, it would have to be a tofu hog, of course). Dr. Jenkins has lots of great data to show that even eating only partially like a Portfolionik will do your cholesterol levels a world of good.

One other dietary bit of advice: in making nutritional adjustments, try to make sure to get your partner onside because the British Family Heart Study found that it's much easier to get people to change their poor health habits if the efforts to change are geared to the couple or family instead of simply to the individual at risk.

As part of a health regimen to lower your cholesterol levels, you may also consider taking all those supplements and nutritional aids that your health-food-nut friends have assured you are bound to save your life and that are reputed to work much better than drugs: stuff like garlic, lecithin, vitamins C and E, and a host of others. These supplements probably do no harm (even though studies have linked higher doses of supplemental vitamin E to a slightly higher risk of premature death) but they are also very unlikely to do you much good. None of these supplements, not a single one, has ever been conclusively linked to a lower risk of heart attack and death from heart attack, not even those delicious (I lie) albeit otherwise beneficial fish oil capsules. Fish, after all, are very complicated animals, and surely when God put them together, She meant for you to eat the whole carp or pike and not to just extract some fatty juice from its skin and meat. Also remember that taking supplements and nutritional aids does not replace the need to make all those other lifestyle adjustments you know you should make, such as:

- stopping smoking
- consulting your doctor about starting an exercise program
- working on reducing your stress levels

And for those of you who figure that "Hey, I don't have to do any of this because drugs and other therapies will do the work for me," I'm afraid not. Drugs have their place but nothing replaces a healthier lifestyle in reducing your risk of heart disease. In fact, one huge review of the benefits of lifestyle versus the benefits of cardiological interventions over the past four decades determined that lifestyle adjustments produced gains up to four times higher in "life-years" than did the best cardiological treatments.

After you have made the aforementioned adjustments in an effort to improve your cholesterol levels, you will want to get retested. Your levels might have improved, which is great news and means that you won't need drugs—so long, of course, as you keep to that healthier lifestyle (although you should get retested periodically to see if your habits are still keeping your levels in check). If, however, like you, your cholesterol levels have refused to budge much, you will have to talk to your doctor about whether you should start taking ASA regularly (see below) and about whether you should start taking drugs to improve your cholesterol levels. If you both agree that drugs are the best way to go, and these days that's a nearly inevitable conclusion, you must next decide which cholesterol-lowering drug is best for you.

For most of us, one of the statin drugs (Lipitor, Mevacor, Pravachol, Zocor, Crestor, Lescol) will be the first-choice medication. Because so many of us have cholesterol problems, statins have now become among the most studied drugs in history, and the very good news is that statins are very effective at lowering LDL, so effective, in fact, that one of them is now being sold over-the-counter in the UK, a decision that is not without its critics (not only because these drugs can occasionally cause life-threatening complications but also because when people start taking a drug, they often abandon the other even more effective strategies to get their condition under control).

So which one to start with? Any one. A great Canadian study showed that in terms of effectiveness, there is really nothing to choose between when looking at these drugs, so start with the cheapest one or the easiest one to take. Also, if one statin doesn't work well enough, switch to another to see what it can do for you instead.

Statins are also very safe (one study estimated serious side effects occur in one in 35,000 patients), although they can be linked to liver damage, severe muscle damage, and kidney damage.

Please note that the latter two problems should never be ignored because they can be so severe that they lead to death. Thus, anyone on a statin who develops intense pain or any changes in the urine must consult a doctor ASAP. (Reports have linked the statin Crestor to a slightly higher risk of these problems, and perhaps even a higher risk of death, but as this is being written, no one has yet come up with a smoking gun to shoot Crestor down.)

Statins also seem to work long term: the earliest followup studies now reveal that the drugs work for at least ten years without any loss of efficacy, and with no increased risk of long-term damage.

Besides improving cholesterol levels and lowering the risk of heart attack and stroke, statins may also have other equally important beneficial effects. Thus, statin use has been linked to lowered risks of several types of cancer (prostate, pancreas, esophagus, breast, and others), dementia, including Alzheimer's disease, and risk of fracture.

Statins don't work for everyone, of course, so that several other drugs are also available to improve cholesterol levels, each of which has its uses and drawbacks. One of the most interesting findings out there is that when statins alone are not enough, combining a statin and niacin, an age-old therapy for abnormal cholesterol levels, results in spectacular improvements (that is, if you can tolerate niacin, which unfortunately produces uncomfortable side effects in a large proportion of people).

As well, and depending on the other risk factors involved, several studies have found that a combination of a statin, a blood pressure–lowering drug (either a beta blocker or an ACE inhibitor or both) along with ASA can be much more effective than statins alone in lowering the risk of death from heart attack, even for people with "normal" blood pressures (see below). In fact, this combo—ASA, three different blood pressure drugs, and two high cholesterol drugs—works so well that a British doctor has argued that the combination of these six drugs should be marketed as a polypill dispensed freely to just about everyone, which is a clear sign that the Apocalypse really is at hand: drugs for everyone and everyone for six drugs. Needless to say, I disagree. Drugs should only be used when other strategies haven't worked, and then each new drug should be administered on its own merits, and not as a BLT serving.

I really can't leave this discussion without commenting on the controversial debate about "how low is too low?" when it comes to cholesterol levels. Thus, some experts believe that you can never get your cholesterol levels low enough, while other believe that there is a downside to lowering cholesterol levels too drastically, such as, for example, perhaps an increased risk of depression and a consequent increased risk of dying from suicide and homicide. I must admit that I have always been quite partial to this latter link because I figure that if some doctor tried to make me stick to an intense low-cholesterol regimen for life, I would surely kill her or, if I couldn't get at her, I would kill myself.

On the ever-present and much larger "other hand," most studies have not found a link between violent death and cholesterol-lowering therapy, and clearly, in the majority of men with significantly raised cholesterol levels, the benefits obtained by improving their cholesterol levels outweigh any small potential risk of depression. As to how far to go with lowering those levels, that again is up to you. But just to be sure, if you are on cholesterol-lowering medication and it's working well, you and your physician should be vigilant for signs of depression, and your physician should be especially wary if you start displaying any interest in joining a gun club.

High Blood Pressure

High blood pressure (hypertension, to doctors) damages your arteries and raises the risk of many health problems, most notably heart attack, dementia, kidney damage, and especially strokes. In fact, high blood pressure (HBP) is the single most important risk factor for stroke, a complication you really don't want to suffer if you plan on enjoying your senior years teaching your grandchildren all those things you failed to teach your kids. Furthermore, midlife man, it's your blood pressure in midlife, not your blood pressure in old age, that is most involved in raising those aforementioned risks, such as the risk of dementia. So if you don't take charge of your blood pressure now, you have way less chance of enjoying the last third of your life (with the only upside being that you may not even know you're not enjoying it).

What may surprise you to learn, though, is that it's not as easy to determine your blood pressure as you might think. For example, in "white coat hypertension" men experience a spike in blood pressure only when it's taken by a health professional, especially some hurry-up passive-aggressive physician visibly anxious to get to the twenty-four other much sicker people waiting impatiently in his exam rooms. If white coaters get their blood pressure taken by a nice mellow machine, however, or better yet, by an attractive member of the sex they prefer, their blood pressure is often normal. The main lesson from all this is that you should never rely on one abnormal in-office blood pressure reading as an indication for treatment (see below).

What will surprise you even more, I'm sure, is that blood pressure ranges have recently been reassessed and the new consensus will affect lots of readers of this book. Thus, it used to be that the cutoff point between high and normal blood pressure was quite simple and applied to everyone equally: anyone with a blood pressure reading of 140/90 or above was said to have HBP, while anyone with a reading below that was said to have normal blood pressure. Also, it used to be that the second number, the diastolic pressure, was way more important in determining the fallout from HBP than the first number, the systolic pressure.

All that is now out the window. Thus, the systolic pressure is now thought to be more important in determining the risks of complication from HBP than the diastolic pressure. We also know now that some people (diabetics, for example, or those with high cholesterol) are much more at risk than others from even minimally elevated blood pressures levels, so people with other risks for heart disease are considered to be at significantly higher risk from blood pressures above 130/80. In fact, many experts now believe that in heart patients and others at high risk, blood pressure can't ever be lowered enough, so long as the low pressure doesn't lead to its own problems such as dizziness and fainting.

It's best, then, to think of blood pressure not in absolute terms according to the numbers, but as part of a syndrome that leads to higher risks of strokes and other complications, and the more of the other risk factors you have for stroke, the lower your blood pressure should be.

And I'll bet you thought that following stock market gyrations was tough!

So what causes your blood pressure to go up? Although raised blood pressure can occasionally be secondary to other health problems (kidney disease, metabolic illnesses such as hyperthyroidism, the use of some medications), over 90 per cent of hypertension is not linked to other health conditions, and is known in the business as "essential" hypertension (the old joke is that

that's because essentially, we don't know anything about it). Factors that raise the risk of hypertension include all the usual suspects:

- excess weight
- excess alcohol intake
- genetic susceptibility
- smoking (curiously, this link is not as clear cut as you'd think)
- unhealthy diet
- sitting on your behind (although it's often quite difficult to lower blood pressure through exercise alone, it's always worth the effort)

Psychological factors also play a strong role for many men. In fact, the Japanese even have a term for death from overwork (between the Germans and the Japanese, they have a term for everything). It's *karoshi* (something several close relatives of mine will never, ever develop) and it's thought that most men who die of *karoshi* do so because of high blood pressure. But it's not just in Japan that high blood pressure takes such a toll on workers. It's equally true everywhere. A study from Cornell University, for example, concluded that the strain of certain modern jobs in which a worker faces high demands but has little control cause "millions of cases" of high blood pressure in the U.S. Another study of British civil servants found that those working in low-level jobs also had much higher blood pressure levels as a consequence (British civil servants work? Who would have guessed? Certainly no one who's ever needed public service in the UK. My son, who lives in Nottingham, calls England "a fourth world" country). High levels of anxiety and depression in middle age have also been shown to be flags for the development of high blood pressure in the future. Your personality, or lack of one, is also a factor, in that pessimists have higher blood pressure than do optimists, but then if you're a pessimist, I suppose you were probably already expecting that bad news.

Prevention includes all the old standbys:

- watching your weight
- not smoking
- exercising
- keeping your cholesterol levels down
- moderating your alcohol intake
- eating a healthy diet
- reducing your stress load

What amount of weight reduction? How much exercise? What kind of stress reduction? "Whatever works for you," is the answer, and to that end, you might be interested to learn that in a study of older adults, tai chi, the ancient low-intensity Chinese physical activity program, was found to reduce blood pressure nearly as much as did moderate-intensity exercise. One of the side effects of tai chi, however, is that an hour after you've finished the exercise session, you're hungry to do it again.

In terms of dietary changes that might lower blood pressure levels, you should eat a well-balanced diet with lots of fruits and veggies and whole grains and legumes, and you should particularly make sure to get enough potassium because many studies have linked a diet rich in potassium with better blood pressure control. So eat lots of bananas, raisins, and apricots. Calcium intake also seems to help control blood pressure, with some studies linking higher milk intake with better blood pressure levels.

As for salt, the consensus these days (subject to change even before you turn the page) is that although we eat far too much salt in a typical western diet, some of us can get away with it and some of us—the salt-sensitive—cannot, and the latter should limit their salt intake to avoid developing high blood pressure. People who already have high blood pressure, however, should always limit their intake of salt and especially avoid prepared foods, which are overloaded with salt, although most of these folks can probably cook with reasonable amounts of salt.

If you are told that you have high blood pressure, the first thing to do is demand a recount. Have it rechecked at least two more times when you are as relaxed as possible—even talking and crossing your legs can raise your blood pressure. If your blood pressure is high on three or more occasions, and you have shut up while it was being taken, you must then decide if it is high enough to necessitate a lifelong commitment to treatment, which always starts, of course, with lifestyle adjustment. Men can often control minimally elevated blood pressure with lifestyle changes, but very few guys are dedicated or disciplined enough to do this for very long, so they nearly always end up on medications, and the choices they are then faced with represent a virtual cornucopia, for which they have to call on all the high school algebra they ever learned to help them figure out the real risk-benefit ratio of a particular medication and the best dose to use.

Given that there are at least three dozen high blood pressure drugs to choose from, the things to ask your doctor about treatment include at least the following:

- Why this drug?
- What are the side effects?
- What are the potential long-term risks?
- Does this drug interact with other drugs I'm taking?
- How often should I come back to reassess my condition?

Also, bear in mind that although there are many new and very powerful and supposedly superior blood pressure drugs on the market now, many of the studies that have shown a clear benefit from lowering blood pressure involved the use of older—and much cheaper—medications, such as diuretics.

Also, get yourself a home blood pressure monitor and use it often. Most studies find that home monitoring is a more accurate measure of what's really happening than occasional stress-provoking measurements in a physician's office.

Finally, taking medications for high blood pressure is often a lifelong commitment, and like other such permanent commitments that end up lasting only a few years, this one needs to be re-evaluated every so often. Up to 30 per cent of older people with high blood pressure can gradually withdraw from medication, and if older people can do it, why not younger ones too? Even if you stop taking medication, however, you should continue to get your blood pressure checked regularly.

Other Risk Factors

Let me get the easy part out of the way quickly—namely, the effect of physical stress on the risk of heart attack. An American study found that in previously largely sedentary men (and any men who are primarily sedentary are usually also large), sudden bursts of activity such as mowing the lawn or shovelling snow can lead to sudden death from the rupture of a plaque on the walls of a sick coronary artery. What should scare many of you is that this type of sudden death seems to happen mostly to men in their fifties. Well, younger and older men are too smart and too lazy to shovel snow. They get someone else to do it for them.

So if sudden bursts of heavy exertion can cause a heart attack, that no doubt immediately brings up the question in most men's minds, and their wives' minds too, I'm sure, what about sex? Sex can kill, I'm afraid, but it should not be your major worry. Although sexual intercourse does slightly increase one's risk of a heart attack, the chance that any individual sex act might set off a heart attack has been estimated to be about one in a million. The mind boggles at some findings. I mean, do you think the researchers went up to guys being resuscitated in the emergency room and asked, "Excuse me, sir, but were you having sex just before you keeled over? Sir? Sir?" And this risk remains higher for about two hours after the sex act. In other words, it's a two-hour-and-three-minute total risk for most men.

Probably of greater worry to us aging men is that this study also found that 10 per cent of heart attacks are triggered by simply rising from sleep in the morning. And no, I'm afraid that my son's solution of staying in bed until the afternoon is not the way to deal with this finding.

Now for the much harder part: the effect of mental stress on heart attack risk. How bad is mental stress for your heart? Baaaad. Stressful events have been shown to:

- lead to a rise in blood pressure and pulse rate
- cause abnormalities in heart rhythm
- cause platelets (blood cells vital in clotting) to become stickier and thus to clot more easily
- produce cardiac ischemia, or decreased blood flow to heart tissue

No wonder, then, that acute and chronic mental stress are both related to a higher risk of heart attack and sudden death, and the higher the stress levels, the more pronounced that effect.. This is something you can (and should) do something about (see Chapter 8).

Moving on to other possible risk factors for heart disease brings us to homocysteine, an amino acid produced from the breakdown of another amino acid, methionine. The best way to lower your homocysteine level is to eat more foods containing vitamins B_{12}, B_6, and folic acid, and that's good advice no matter what role homocysteine may turn out to have or not have in heart disease.

Several studies have also found a link between high iron stores in the body and a higher risk of heart attack, and a study from Kansas University Medical Centre found that donating one unit of blood every three years reduced the risk of a heart attack by 30 per cent. So go ahead and give them a pint every so often. Not only will it allow you to act excessively self-righteous, it might even be good for you. And it will certainly help others.

Perhaps the most intriguing link between heart disease and newer risk factors, and certainly the one getting most attention these days, is the potential one between heart attacks and infections or inflammation in general. For example, studies have linked heart attacks in younger men with an infection with an organism called *Chlamydia pneumoniae,* while several others have linked higher levels of C-reactive protein, or CRP (a measure of inflammation), from gum disease and other chronic inflammatory conditions with a higher risk of heart attack and stroke. So don't get infected. And floss. Next. Actually, before you go, you might consider getting your CRP level checked. Now go.

One final word about heart disease and it's probably the most important advice: don't spend too much time worrying about it. Do the best you can and then get on with your life. According to Dr. James Muller of Deaconess Hospital, Harvard Medical School, who was quoted in *USA Today,* "If a person did everything he could to avoid triggering a heart attack, he'd probably die of boredom."

ASA (Acetylsalicylic Acid) Therapy

Taking ASA every day to prevent heart attack and stroke has proven to be most effective in high-risk men, such as those who have already had a heart attack or those with established coronary heart disease. In lower-risk men, it is likely that daily ASA use also prevents heart attacks but it's still a bit of a hot issue in medical circles, mainly because as men get older, the risks of taking daily ASA (see below) may start to outweigh the benefits.

If you decide to take ASA daily, one problem you run into is that doctors still don't know the best dose. The less you take the better, of course, but only if you take enough of it to do you some good, and that amount can vary for each of us. For example, several studies have determined that some people (perhaps 25 per cent of us) are ASA "resistant," that is, they need higher doses of ASA to get its full anti-clotting effect. So, although it's likely that 81 mg (a baby ASA) is enough for most people, many others need much higher doses to prevent heart attacks, doses at which the complications of ASA are more likely to kick in.

How can you tell if you're ASA resistant? There are tests but they are not used much because there still seems to be a lot of disagreement about how accurate they are, so the first knowledge you may have that the ASA didn't do you any good is when you're looking down from above as they are saying Kaddish over you.

So how do you decide what to do? Well, as always, you don't start by reaching for a bottle, but rather by discussing the pros and cons with your physician. The most important pro is that ASA use lowers the risk of heart attack. Regular use of ASA has also been linked to a lower risk of several types of cancer including colon cancer. And taking nonsteroidal anti-inflammatories (NSAIDS) regularly has been linked to a lower risk of dementia, including the dementia of Alzheimer's disease.

Now for the cons. So why shouldn't every man be taking ASA? Because, as my chummy professors used to yell at me as I headed out the door well before the lecture was over, "Not so quick, you there." (I was always "you there" in medical school, just as I am at home.) The following factors mitigate against taking an ASA every day:

- Some people are allergic to ASA.
- ASA can produce bothersome side effects, most notably gastrointestinal disturbances such as an upset stomach and nausea, a risk that can be lowered but not eliminated by using enteric-coated ASA.
- Regular use of ASA is linked to a significantly higher risk of stomach ulcers, which not only can cause pain but can also bleed and even rupture, a risk that is not reduced by the use of enteric-coated ASA.
- Anyone at risk of a bleeding problem puts himself at even higher risk if he also starts to take ASA regularly, since ASA inhibits clotting. Thus, regular use of ASA increases the risk of dying from a cerebral hemorrhage due to a ruptured blood vessel in the brain (this accounts for about 20 per cent of all strokes).
- Finally, a recent study questioned the effectiveness of taking ASA in conjunction with NSAIDS such as naproxen and ibuprofen, something that millions of ASA users do. It's a small study that suggests further research is needed, but it found that in some people the anti-clotting effect of ASA is lowered by the concomitant use of other NSAIDS.

So it's clearly not a one-size-fits-all formula. As with so many other medical issues, you must weigh the pros and cons of this issue and decide for yourself.

Finally, one situation that demands the immediate use of ASA is when you think you are having a heart attack or simply feel that you're in imminent danger of having one, such as coming home to find your wife gone, your house bare, and a note on the floor with your name on it. Downing a prophylactic ASA immediately in those situations can save your life by preventing a blood clot from forming in the first place or by preventing a small clot from getting larger. It won't bring back the couch or lamps (Hey! Did you ever really notice them before anyway?), but it will better your chances to live and fight in court another day.

Osteoarthritis

Rheumatologists recognize over one hundred forms of arthritis (I have no idea how many they can't recognize), but the only one I want to discuss is osteoarthritis (OA), or degenerative arthritis, which is showing up with increasing frequency in middle-aged adults, often as a result of all that pounding of pavement younger runners did when the mantra was "No pain, no gain." Well, that mantra, like so many others (don't trust anyone over thirty; socialism is the wave of the future; the UN will usher in an era of world peace) was wrong and baby boomers in their forties and fifties are now paying the price, queuing up in ever-larger numbers for replacement hips and knees. That said, osteoarthritis goes up dramatically with age, so that over 70 per cent of adults over the age of sixty have some degree of OA, produced by deterioration in the articular cartilage in a joint, the cartilage that cushions movement between bones. No wonder, then, that the major symptoms of OA are pain, stiffness, crackling sounds in the joint, and joint swelling.

The joints most commonly affected by OA are the weight-bearing ones, such as the knees and hips, as well as those in the spine and thumbs. Osteoarthritis of the knee is one of the leading causes of disability in elderly North Americans, and the risk of getting it goes up directly with weight. A study of physicians found that the heavier a guy is in his younger years (read: now), the greater his eventual risk of OA of the hip or knee (read: soon). Other factors that increase the risk of OA are a family history of degenerative arthritis, injury to the joint, malalignment of the bones, a history of cartilage or ligament tear, and calcium deposits or other inflammation in or around the joint.

Once again, treatment starts with prevention. So never get injured. You're welcome. What is perhaps more feasible is to avoid excess weight, and if you are already overweight, to lose as many of those excess pounds as you can, although I don't think that if OA affects your thumb losing weight is nearly as important as when it affects your knee or back. In addition, a recent study claims that elite athletes seem to have a higher risk of degenerative arthritis, but somehow I don't think that's going to matter much to too many of my readers.

When it comes to treating OA, exercise is, as always, numero uno, which may be a surprise to some of you, given that exercise increases the pain of OA. But it's quite clear that exercise not only improves physical performance, it also lessens pain and slows the natural progress of OA. And although it's often hard to do exercise when your joints hurt a lot with every movement, if you can limit the pain with some analgesics or NSAIDS (see below), you will be able to do more, which will lessen your eventual pain and slow the deterioration of that joint. So you want to do as much as you can. To gauge how much that is, first figure out which activities trigger your pain and how much of each trigger is required for the pain to set in. Then try to adjust your pain-control strategies to minimize the effects of that trigger. So, for example, if your daily three-mile walk always sets off enough pain to require you to take medication afterwards, you might try taking an NSAID or acetaminophen as a prophylactic measure before the walk. This doesn't mean that you put a condom on when you set out; it means that you take the pill *before* starting the activity, which may lessen your need for even more medication afterwards, and may allow you to do more exercise while you're walking.

Other strategies you may want to try include a diet high in fish oils, which has been linked to less joint inflammation (even though inflammation is not a major component of OA, it's still worth a try because two or three trout sure tops tons of Tylenol). In addition, the multifaceted Framingham Study, which has been charting the health of the citizens of Framingham, Massachusetts, for nearly five decades, has revealed that a diet high in vitamins C and D, meaning a diet high in fruits and veggies, is linked to a lower risk of osteoarthritis and a slower rate of progression of existing OA. Other standard therapies for osteoarthritis include some form of physical treatment, such as physiotherapy, as well as analgesics such as acetaminophen, ASA and other NSAID medications, COX-2 inhibitors such as celecoxib (Celebrex), and sometimes even cortisone.

If you have to take NSAIDS or COX-2 inhibitors, always keep in mind that these are drugs with significant risks, and those risks often outweigh the benefits. The most important risk associated with the use of NSAIDS is gastric bleeding. These drugs not only irritate the stomach, producing such common side effects as heartburn and abdominal pain, they actually erode the stomach lining, which can lead to potentially life-threatening complications such as ulcers and stomach rupture. Since NSAIDS do not always produce noticeable symptoms while eroding the stomach lining, some people die of a ruptured ulcer without ever having known they were developing the problem, so don't just assume that "no symptoms means no problems." With an NSAID (as with any drug), always use the weakest formulation and lowest dose of that drug for the least amount of time you can get away with. And since these drugs do not in any way alter the course of OA but merely control some of the symptoms, always try to get away from using these drugs altogether, if possible. But if you do have to use one for a long time and in high doses, you should talk to your doctor about the advisability of taking a stomach-protecting drug such as misoprostol along with the NSAID.

And then, there's the risk of heart attack and stroke. Several very large studies have now confirmed that both NSAIDS and COX-2 inhibitors (which are promoted largely because they are said to cause less stomach irritation and hence lead to a lower risk of bleeding and ulcer than do NSAIDS), raise the risk of heart attack and stroke. As I write this, the jury is still out on how significant that risk is, at what dose it kicks in, and how long you have to be on the pills to experience that higher risk. If you ask me, though, I think that any increased risk at all is probably not worth it for the vast majority of people who use these drugs, which, after all, do not alter the course of any condition but simply alleviate some symptoms—maybe.

So, as with NSAIDS, if you have to use a COX-2 inhibitor, I caution you to 1) continually weigh and re-evaluate the risks against the over-touted benefits, and 2) to use the lowest dose of the weakest formulation for the least amount of time possible. And if you're at particularly high risk for heart attack anyway, you might want to be very prudent in your use of any of these drugs—yes, even in the short term.

Many people with OA swear by glucosamine and chondroitin sulfate, two natural substances involved in the formation of cartilage that have long been used in animals and in Europe (no connection there as far as I can tell) because these two substances are said to rebuild joint cartilage. Although there is no proof that they actually do that, there is some empirical evidence that glucosamine and chondroitin sulfate can decrease pain in joints affected with osteoarthritis, and since there seems to be little downside to either, I really don't see why you wouldn't try them.

In lab studies, doxycycline, a member of the tetracycline family, has been shown to block the enzymes involved in cartilage breakdown, and although this work is now over a decade old, there is still no confirmation that doxycycline is useful in OA. Stay tuned, though.

One thing you shouldn't do for your joint pain is move somewhere with a warmer climate, such as Arizona or California. For years, doctors in Montreal, where I first practised, used to tell their complaining arthritic patients, "Oy! Morris! If you could just move to Arizona, Morris, you would be so much better. Arizona, Morris. That's where you should move, and believe me, your pain will be gone. Abi gezunt!" Why? Because the doctor knew that even if the move didn't help Morris, at least the doctor's discomfort would improve the instant Morris toted his tush to Tucson. But according to a study in the journal *Pain,* there really is no one best climate for arthritis. Weather, this study found, affects people's perception of pain no matter where they live, so the best thing to do is to sit tight and continue to kvetch at home.

Osteoporosis

Osteoporosis (OP) is a men's disease. Too. Sure, OP hits more women, but about 20 per cent of all OP patients are men, and one-third of all hip fractures occur in men. Not only that, when men do fracture a hip, they tend to do much more poorly than women in large part because men with fractured hips tend to be older and sicker specimens. And in case you think, as Dooley Wilson had it in *Casablanca,* that a hip is just a hip, think again because at least one-third of men who break their hips die within a year of the fracture, and 50 per cent of the others never regain their full mobility. That's a hell of a price to pay for a disease that may be largely preventable.

It's not just broken hips that should make you wary of OP, either. Osteoporosis also affects the spine and leads to fractures in the spinal column and the bones of the wrist. (Boy! Did we ever see lots of those on icy days in Montreal, which occur from early October to late June: you gotta love that city—indoors.) Spinal column fractures not only cause a great deal of pain but also produce a consequent loss of height with age, a sobering prospect for a man of five foot six like me, or at least it used to be five foot six.

The risk factors for osteoporosis are generally the same in men as in women:

- getting older
- being of European or Asian descent
- being a smoker
- abusing alcohol
- living a largely sedentary lifestyle
- having a strong family history of osteoporosis
- taking in too little calcium and vitamin D (vitamin D helps calcium get absorbed)
- taking in too much vitamin A
- having low testosterone levels
- using certain drugs, including steroids, thyroid hormone, and anticonvulsants
- having a very high protein intake
- eating a high-salt diet

- having certain chronic conditions, including hyperthyroidism, hyperparathyroidism, celiac disease (le celiac, c'est moi), a host of gastrointestinal illnesses, epilepsy, and other neurologic conditions

OP is best prevented if you start early in life. That's because bones are like bank accounts: the more you can store in them when you're young, the more you have to draw on when they inevitably shrink with age. Thus, to build a healthy bone bank kids must get enough calcium and vitamin D and, more important, do enough weight-bearing exercise in the first twenty-five years of life. After that, I'm sorry to say, your bone bank account is as thick as it's going to get and after the age of thirty or so, bones start to thin, slowly at first, much more rapidly later on.

You can significantly retard the rate of bone loss by:

- doing weight-bearing exercise—activities such as jogging, walking, and resistance training; anything involving jumping is great, but only, of course, if you live on the ground floor
- not smoking
- limiting your alcohol intake to moderate amounts
- consuming enough calcium and vitamin D (although I don't think you need to make a fetish of ensuring that you get the exact recommended daily intake of 1,200 to 1,500 mg)

High-calcium foods include dairy products, broccoli, tofu, beans, shrimp, sardines, and salmon bones, and an interesting recent study also linked a compound in onions with reduced bone thinning, although I doubt that you'll stick with this diet for very long if it means sitting down to a daily evening meal of soy cubes, sardines, salmon bones, onions, and beans (at the very least, your family will quickly abandon you). For those of you who can't stand or can't ingest dairy products and who thus rely on calcium-fortified foods such as OJ, an interesting study found that calcium-fortified foods may not be as rich a source of calcium as you may think. In this study, the amount of calcium that was absorbed from two different orange juices fortified with calcium varied significantly among a group of volunteers. "OJ guilty," I think the headline read.

When it comes to calcium supplements, take the kind that best suits you and your pocketbook, although calcium citrate is probably less likely to cause stomach upsets than calcium carbonate. Also, for best absorption, try to take the supplements on an empty stomach, and also keep in mind that calcium supplements can interfere with the absorption of some other medications you may be taking. But no matter which form you take, you should also be sure to get enough vitamin D with your calcium by getting some sun exposure (ten minutes a day is probably enough). If you live in a city like Vancouver, however, getting that amount of sunshine is impossible eleven months a year, so you might prefer to eat more vitamin D–enriched foods or better yet, I think, to take vitamin D supplements. By the way, my mom swears that the easiest and cheapest way to get enough calcium is to take four or five Tums a day, and although I can't comment about the "easiest" part, I bet you she's right about the "cheapest" part. That's one area where that woman has never been wrong.

Periodontal Disease

Like many people my age, I have developed periodontal disease, a chronic, persistent, and (in my severe case) often painful inflammation of the gums and supporting structures of the teeth.

The earliest stage of periodontal disease is gingivitis, an inflammation caused by the buildup of gunk, which dentists, who are often frustrated doctors, have taken to calling plaque. This is not, please note, the same kind of plaque that hits your arteries and which doctors take care of (although I wish that cleaning an artery were as simple as flossing it a few times a week). Depending on its severity, periodontal disease produces such symptoms as bleeding, swollen, red, and tender gums, as well as bad breath and a bad taste in the mouth. If allowed to proceed unchecked, periodontal disease leads to gum recession, loose teeth, and "tilting" of the teeth, which is why periodontal disease has become the most common cause of tooth loss in people over the age of forty. In fact, my periodontist is fond of telling me as I lie back in his chair, captive and rubber-dammed, "You know, your teeth are in great shape, Art. It's your gums that will have to come out. Ha, ha. Open wider."

More significant than lost teeth, though, is the fact that periodontal disease has been linked to much higher risks of heart disease and stroke and perhaps even dementia. How can plaque on your gums (which is really nothing more than oral schmutz, after all) have anything to do with plaque on your arteries (which consists of inflammatory material, calcium, cholesterol, blood cells, and other stuff) or even plaque in your brain? The common link is thought to be inflammation (see heart disease—above), so that inflammation anywhere in the body, even in your yellowed gums, produces inflammatory proteins, which in turn, some experts believe, induce inflammation elsewhere, such as in coronary arteries and brain tissue. Bottom line: as my unfunny dentist loves to remind me, "Floss or die, Art. Floss or die. My dental hygienist will see you now for about thirty minutes and after that my dental money-taker will rob you of 110 dollars. Have a nice day."

The treatment for periodontal disease is proper dental care, regular flossing and cleaning, and occasionally, antibiotics to kill the bacteria. Perhaps the most important aspect of treatment, though, is to try to find a periodontist who is actually funny, a task akin to locating the Holy Grail.

Stroke

You should familiarize yourself with how to recognize the signs of a stroke, although I sincerely hope you never have to use this information.

There are two reasons for this. First, there is excellent evidence that small strokes or mini-strokes (what doctors call TIAS for transient ischemic attacks) are really only strokes-in-waiting, so if you suffer any of the symptoms listed below, you must make sure to see a doctor ASAP, even if the symptoms are transient. If you don't take care of things, you remain at much higher risk of suffering a full-blown stroke both in the near and distant future.

Also, we now know that quickly treating the most common kind of strokes, the ones caused by blockage in the arterial supply to a part of the brain, can not only limit some of the damage that the stroke is set to produce, much as treating a heart attack within several hours can result in saving much heart tissue, but quick treatment can, in some circumstances, even reverse the damage resulting from the stroke.

Unhappily, however, the public is just not getting the message. Thus, a majority of people at increased risk for a stroke are unaware of their risk, and in one study, only about 25 per cent of stroke patients correctly identified their symptoms as stroke-related—that is, 75 per cent did not know that what they were suffering was a stroke. So it's no great surprise that a large majority of people who could benefit from anti-stroke therapy do not make it to the hospital in the six-hour window of opportunity for intervention.

This is especially important information, then, for those at high risk of stroke, especially anyone with:

- atrial fibrillation (an abnormal heart rhythm)
- high blood pressure
- heart disease

- risk factors for heart disease such as high cholesterol, sedentary lifestyle, and obesity
- narrowed carotid arteries
- a previous TIA or stroke
- a history of blood clots

So put this in your "can't forget" memory compartment. If you can't remember where that is, ask your wife. She'll know for sure. Symptoms that require immediate attention include:

- sudden weakness or paralysis in a limb or facial muscles on one side of the body
- sudden difficulty speaking or understanding speech (except, I suppose, when listening to sports announcers)
- sudden loss of vision
- sudden extreme dizziness or loss of balance, especially when it's associated with one of the other signs
- a sudden very severe headache (not your usual migraine but the kind of headache that is described as the worst you've ever had)

All these symptoms should be treated as an extreme emergency (yes, there are grades of emergency—just ask any Canadian sitting for eighteen hours in a hospital ER). Drop everything (you may have no choice) and call 9-1-1 for an ambulance. Do not drive yourself to the ER and don't call your Aunt Emily's nanny to come get you. Get the ambulance to siren you to an ER where you can be evaluated. Happily, many times, the cause of these symptoms will not be a stroke, but never take that chance. Hey, I want you around to read my other books.

{6}

PLAN A: YOU ARE WHAT YOU EAT AND DRINK

• • •

If I had known that I was going to live this long,
I would have taken better care of myself.

MICKEY MANTLE

Not only do persons with better health
habits survive longer, disability is postponed and
compressed into fewer years at the end of life.

ANTHONY J. VITA, ET AL., *New England Journal of Medicine*

Trying in my usual gentle manner to make a point one day, I asked one of the nonmedical reviewers of this text if he had been struck by the connection among the chronic health problems discussed in the preceding chapter. The immediate reply was, "Sure, man. They're all things that only happen to you when you're really old. Like over fifty." Not for the first time did it occur to me that things might work much better if teenage sons and their fathers inhabited separate planets.

"No," I persisted. "What I meant is that all those diseases are nearly entirely preventable if you do all the right things starting early in life."

"There you go again, man," came the reply. "As usual, you're trying to turn everything into a lecture. I'm outta here, man."

"Man"? Whatever happened to "Dad"? And lecture? Hey, gimme a break. Is that what this really reads like, I wondered for a nanosecond before dismissing his clearly inaccurate assessment and banning that boy from using the car for a month. But his words do lead me to make this disclaimer: none of this should read like a lecture for the simple reason that lectures about lifestyle never alter behaviour. All I am aiming to do is point out how the choices you have already made might affect you, and after you pick yourself up off the floor from that fright, I want to let you know what you can now do to minimize your health risks, and when I'm done, you can decide what to do with that information. But remember, no soup for you if you don't listen to at least some of what I say.

So let me start by telling you that an interesting study in the *Journal of the American Medical Association* concluded that death in old age is never the result of only one cause. Rather, we tend to die as a result of several underlying factors that are generally a product of "lifelong habits," nearly all of which can largely be changed.

The good news is that we are getting the message—to a certain extent. And happily, guys, men may be getting the message more clearly than women. As proof, there's the narrowing mortality gap between men and women. You see, in most western countries and most cultures women have been outliving men by an average of seven to eight years, a gap that has remained pretty consistent for about a hundred years.

Why do men die so much sooner than women? No one really knows, although of the fifteen leading causes of death, men are number one in all of them, and of the seventy-two leading causes of death in North America, women have a higher death rate from only six of them: breast cancer (pretty clear why), pregnancy and childbirth (ditto), Alzheimer's disease (well, women have smaller brains to begin with, oops!), asthma, rheumatic fever, and kidney infections.

By the way, whenever I give a talk about healthy lifestyle, I always ask the audience for ideas about why women outlive men. When I posed this question to one audience, a woman in her senior years sitting next to her very sour-looking and irascible husband, instantly shot her hand up and offered, "Because we deserve to." Just as the laughter was dying down, the gent looked over at his mate and boomed, "Well, we want to die first."

Anyway, there are a host of potential reasons for this difference in mortality—hormones (estrogen protects, testosterone kills?), women sleep better and deal with stress better than men, women have less dangerous jobs, women use support services and social contacts and medical intervention more wisely than men do (for example, deaths from melanoma are 50 per cent higher in men, although men tend to suffer 50 per cent fewer melanomas than women)—but one factor that has clearly played a role is differences in lifestyle. In the past, women may have had somewhat healthier lifestyles than men, although that may be changing with all the young women who are smoking now and with more men taking better care of themselves.

In fact, happily for Canadian men, that decades-long seven-year gap in life expectancy between men and women in Canada has now shrunk to less than five years, in part because men's improved lifestyles have resulted in a more rapid decrease in deaths from heart attacks and strokes than has been seen among women.

In case any of you guys are tempted to rest on your laurels, however, don't, because we could still be doing much better. Although we're living longer, we're also spending more time on the disabled list. Thus, a UK report shows that time spent disabled by disease has risen for men by 34 per cent since 1981, no surprise, really, when you consider that a recent study found that only 3 per cent of adults are acting on all four of the key injunctions for healthy living: not smoking, eating at least five servings of fruits and veggies a day, exercising thirty minutes a day for most days of the week, and maintaining a BMI under 25 (see below).

So this chapter and the next two are devoted to trying to get you to change to a more healthy lifestyle because, according to a study in the *New England Journal of Medicine,* "Not only do persons with better health habits survive longer, disability is postponed and compressed into fewer years at the end of life." And hey, don't you want to live longer with less time spent disabled? If you don't, you can skip to Chapter 9.

An important caveat, however. As you will quickly notice, I have been very selective in the healthy lifestyle habits that I've chosen to cover. Thus, I will not discuss the need to avoid too much sun exposure (self-evident, although be aware that a little sun exposure—ten to fifteen minutes a day—is not only desirable, it may even be necessary to maintain adequate vitamin D levels) or the hazards of recreational drug use (hey, dude, don't do 'em). I discuss only what I consider to be the most important healthy lifestyle habits that affect most of us. You will notice, too, that I have divided my advice about health into three chapters. This chapter discusses things you should and should not ingest; the next deals with weight control, exercise, and other aspects of healthy living; and the following chapter deals with aspects of psychological health—treating depression and handling stress.

Diet

Most of you eat too much, and this not only makes you fat, it may also be leading you to an earlier death (gulp!). For example, in some very famous experiments, when researchers reduced the food intake of lab rats and mice by 30 to 40 per cent, the rats and mice extended their life spans by about one-third. What is true for rodents is probably also true for humans (although as any careful researcher will point out, people are not simply large mice or rats, except, of course, for my lawyer). Thus, we have some preliminary data to show that calorie restriction in humans correlates with less heart disease and slower neurological deterioration. According to no less an authority than the *New England Journal of Medicine,* "calorie restriction slows age-related deficits in behavior, learning, immune response, gene expression, and DNA repair," a lot of deficits you would really like to avoid because they shorten your life expectancy and increase the number of health problems you come down with. Indeed, calorie restriction is now so hyped as a key to longer and better life that several hundred idiots, excuse me, several hundred well-informed health consumers (often the same thing), are literally starving themselves (averaging fewer than 1,000 calories a day, 24/7) in an attempt to live longer. "Morons," my son opined while chomping on a hot dog. "Quite agree, quite agree," I concurred through bites of my own.

Those idiots may be extremists but they do make the point that you can live a very healthy life eating a whole lot less, and so you should. And you can start by limiting your portions. Portion size has exploded in North America, along with our waistlines, and these two phenomena are intimately connected. Thus, studies have shown that the more you put on someone's plate, the more he eats. We are, after all, well-bred boys and girls brought up to finish every morsel because if we don't, as our mothers relentlessly explained, a kid in China is going to starve. How that kid ever knew that I wasn't mopping up all my sauce, I never figured out, but I mopped away just in case. Portion size is so important in how much we eat that one study has even shown that if you just serve food on smaller plates, people eat less.

Most of you also don't eat regularly enough, even though what Mom told you is really true: eating three meals a day with small healthy snacks in between is important, although if I had to single out one meal for emphasis, that one would clearly be breakfast, which not only sets the metabolic table for the rest of the day but also helps you limit how much you eat the rest of the day. For example, a British study found that people who eat breakfast with some cereal in it tend to eat fewer fatty foods the rest of the day, and thus control their weights better. As empirical proof, a survey of over thirty thousand people who have lost considerable amounts of weight and who have managed to keep it off for many years found that one of the common denominators for such people is eating a good breakfast regularly. Another study on obese kids found the same thing: the better the breakfast, the less they ate throughout the day.

But it's not just in maintaining healthy weight that eating breakfast is important. A good breakfast also leads to better health. British researchers, for example, claim that breakfast eaters tend to get a healthy serving of vital fibre and vitamins from their breakfast foods, although they clearly did not mean those who eat the typical British breakfast of three fried eggs, sausage, bacon, kippers, fried tomato, and that acme of British cuisine, fried bread. Eating breakfast has also been shown to lead to less insulin resistance and hence lowered risks of developing diabetes and its attendant complications.

Breakfast also helps your brain. Thus, several studies have shown that students score better on cognitive and memory tests on the days they eat breakfast compared with the days they skip breakfast. They are also more alert and attentive in class after eating breakfast. And seniors who eat breakfast regularly score better on cognitive tests, too, such as remembering to take their prunes.

Bottom line: eat a healthy breakfast every day. I, for example, now consume a breakfast that consists of a bowl of gluten-free, unsweetened cereal, mixed with a large serving of blueberries (I freeze bags of fresh blueberries in the summer when they're cheap. Hey, I'm my mother's son.), and often with half a sliced banana. It's not only a delicious way to start the day, it also allows me to snack less than I used to do.

Most of you also don't eat slowly enough. Your mother was right in this, too, guys. Eating more slowly has been linked to several health benefits, the most interesting one being a lower risk of obesity. That's right, a study of twenty-eight overweight men and women found that the slower the study participants ate, the less they tended to take in.

Most of us also eat too much of the wrong foods and don't eat enough of the right ones, which is partly why North America is experiencing an epidemic of heart disease, stroke, diabetes, even cancer. An international panel of experts has claimed that 30 to 40 per cent of all cancers could be avoided if people ate a healthier diet and got enough exercise.

What kind of foods am I talking about? Simple. On the one hand, we ingest too much:

- protein (this is one thing your mom was wrong about; most of us don't really need to worry about how much protein we're getting)
- sugar

- refined carbohydrates
- saturated fat, especially the kind found in red meat (although there's a debate developing about whether all saturated fats are equally harmful)
- trans fat, which is found mostly in fast foods and prepared foods, and which I believe is the worst of the "bad fat lot" (so if you make only one change to your diet after reading this section, cut down on your intake of trans fat)
- salt
- carbonated beverages

On the other hand, we don't eat enough:

- fruits and veggies of all kinds
- fish (but only baked or broiled fish; fishsticks are not fish—I don't know what they are, but I can say I've never seen a fishstick swimming in the sea or a tank)
- legumes
- fibre
- monounsaturated fats

The great news is that the best way to get more of those foods into you is easy, fun, and delicious. It goes by many names and guises (depending on which foods are stressed), but the name I favour and the one used most often is the Mediterranean diet, which stresses a limited intake of meat and a high intake of fruits, veggies, beans, fish, some grains, small amounts of cheese and yogurt, and foods rich in monounsaturated fats, especially olives. Many well-designed, long-term studies have shown conclusively that people who follow a Med-fed diet tend to die at significantly slower rates and develop many degenerative diseases much more slowly than people who eat a standard western-style diet with its emphasis on meat, meat, meat, meat, fries, meat, meat, meat, and ice cream. For example, one study of 1,300 adults with heart disease found that those who followed a Mediterranean diet most closely were 30 per cent more likely to be alive after four years than those who didn't.

And if you switch to a Mediterranean diet, the great news is that it doesn't take long to get the benefits. In the most stark example of how quickly it can make a difference, heart attack victims who switched to a Mediterranean diet lowered the risk of a second heart attack by over 75 per cent over two years compared with people who continued to eat as before.

Bottom line: if you're a typical North American male, you probably need to eat way more fruits and veggies and fish and whole grains and legumes, including beans (the latter, though, should be introduced slowly into the diet, for reasons of family closeness).

I know, however, that no matter what the evidence shows and no matter how much I exhort you, many of you will find it very difficult to abandon your prime rib and baked potato with sour cream for baked breast of tofu and low-fat yogurt. So here's something to chew on, guys. Take your time. There's no great rush to change. You've taken fifty years to become what you are, so what's the big deal if it takes you a year or two to undo some of the damage. It's easier to do this if you go about it slowly (remember those beans). And you're more likely to stick with it if you don't do it precipitously.

Rather, make one or two small adjustments at a time (starting with say, two extra servings of veggies a day) and then when you have arrived at a satisfactory diet, one that should make you both healthy and happy, stop there. You don't really have to push it all the way to becoming a vegetarian or (horrors!) a vegan, even if a vegetarian diet is generally very healthy. If you ask me, though, a vegetarian diet has a lot going against it. First, most people who set out to become vegetarians don't stick with it for very long. It's OK for teenagers who want to upset their parents. When they hit college, however, burgers will nearly always beat out beans for big meals out.

Second, although vegetarians don't die as much from heart disease and cancer, they are much more likely than meat eaters to die of boredom. (After all, how many different recipes can you come up with for a zucchini casserole?)

Third, a vegetarian diet may not be what evolution had in mind for you. According to one theory, the move away from a vegetarian diet is what allowed our ancestors' brains to grow, or to put it in pictures, it wasn't an apple the snake gave Eve, it was a pepperoni. This theory postulates that once they were freed of the need to use so much energy to digest the vast amounts of rabbit food necessary to stem their hunger, early man and woman were able to devote more energy to thinking. ("Why are we eating grass when we could have foie gras, Thor?") Thus, meat eaters became wiser and were able to avoid becoming prey, while vegetarians continued to be eaten by predators no matter how much they prayed. Interestingly but not surprisingly, vegetarians may still be as dumb as they were back then, which is what may account for an American survey that found self-proclaimed vegetarians reported eating more fish and poultry over a two-week test period than did self-proclaimed carnivores.

So if you want to start slowly, which of those ingredients of a Mediterranean diet should you stress? I would certainly start by increasing my intake of fruits and particularly veggies. Veggies and fruits are easy to add into a diet—"any idiot can make a salad," says my wife, "even you"—and they contain so many vital elements, such as fibre, complex carbohydrates, minerals, especially rich supplies of antioxidants (flavonoids, sulforophane, phenols, quercetin, and dozens more) and antioxidant vitamins (vitamins C, E, folic acid, beta-carotene, etc.). Antioxidants are the flavour-du-jour these days because they mop up harmful chemicals called free radicals, those dirty little Abby Hoffmans that are produced by oxygenation reactions in the body and that lead to degenerative diseases and aging. But there's also this to recommend more fruits and veggies: filling up on salad and such lowers your intake of other less healthy foods.

Next, I would focus on eating more fish, especially oily fish, such as salmon. Fish are loaded with minerals, antioxidants, vitamins (vitamin D, for example, which is hard to get naturally from food sources), and especially healthy oils. So it's no wonder, I suppose, that those Japanese who never eat fish (apparently there are some somewhere) were found to have a 32 per cent higher mortality rate than those who eat fish daily, and those numbers would be even more in favour of the fish eaters, I think, if the Japanese didn't also have a nasty habit of eating fish and fish products (like fugu) that can kill you instantly. (My son has a theory that whatever we non-Japanese view as disgusting, the Japanese consider a delicacy, and I have not yet been able to prove him wrong.)

Since fish also has a strong anti-inflammatory effect, eating more fish can help with all sorts of health problems such as heart disease, depression, arthritis, asthma, perhaps even with lowering the risk of some kinds of dementia. And don't be put off by the outcry about the high mercury levels in fish. Yes, kids and women in childbearing years should be careful about the amount of mercury they consume from fish, but as a midlife man, you're neither a kid nor a childbearing female, so eat all the fish you like, although if you start glowing green at night, then cut back on the tuna a bit.

Next, I would try to increase my intake of whole grains and beans, not only because of their mineral and vitamin and antioxidant load but also because of their high fibre content, since a high fibre intake is associated with lower risks of many common illnesses linked to our western way of life, such as:

- obesity
- heart disease
- Type II diabetes
- high blood pressure
- gastrointestinal problems such as gallstones, appendicitis, irritable bowel syndrome, hemorrhoids, and diverticulosis
- colon polyps and colon cancer
- other cancers

Another food group that I particularly like is dairy products, especially cheese and yogurt, mostly because dairy products are delicious treats. I can't cite any studies proving that you live longer if you eat lots of cheese, but I can certainly attest that you will enjoy your life much more if you regularly sup on gobs of feta, fresh mozzarella, dauphin, old cheddar, and so on.

But there's also that calcium you get from dairy products. Now, most experts stress taking in lots of calcium to prevent osteoporosis and bone fractures (see Chapter 5). I must say, however, that I'm not convinced that loading up on calcium is nearly as important in maintaining healthy bones in aging people as most experts feel it is. So while I do believe that eating lots of calcium-rich foods is vital in kids and young adults to help them build bone mass, if you want to maintain that bone mass, I think it's more important to do lots of weight-bearing exercise than it is to drink lots of milk. That said, there is very little downside to eating lots of calcium-rich foods (except perhaps for a slightly raised increased risk of prostate cancer and kidney stones) and there may be quite an upside. A higher intake of calcium has been linked to better weight control (see Chapter 7), lower blood pressure, and lower rates of some cancers. No surprise, then, that a study that followed several hundred Welsh men for twenty years (the researchers must have had to endure endless hours of choral music) found that those men who drank the most milk had the lowest overall rate of death when compared with men who drank the least milk. I don't know that milk helps you live longer (other factors could have affected the outcome in this study) but it certainly doesn't seem to lead to higher rates of death from heart attack and stroke as is commonly feared. If I were loading up on lots of milk, however, I would favour skim milk or reduced fat milk. And if you do eat lots of calcium to protect your bones, remember this: it does you little good if you don't also take in extra vitamin D.

You should also introduce far more monounsaturated fats to your diet, starting by cooking with olive oil, and by eating a variety of nuts—almonds, cashews, peanuts, macadmias, pecans—whatever you like and can afford. I also would encourage you to eat snacks of nuts and berries. These are not only exceedingly healthy foods, they can help curb your appetite. I find that a regular small snack of my famous trail mix consisting of almonds, cashews, peanuts, raisins or currants, sunflower or pumpkin seeds, and definitely cranberries (which are now said to help you fight viruses, too), always takes the edge off my ever-present peckishness, and I firmly believe that eating trail mix regularly is what has most helped me keep off the thirty-five pounds I lost six years ago (that, and the threat of a divorce from my wife should I ever gain those pounds back).

Finally, if you don't think you can get enough good fats from olives and avocados and nuts, why not add in some good quality dark chocolate, which has loads of antioxidants in it? It's not on most experts' list of foods that make up a Mediterranean diet, but it sure is on mine, as is regular intake of moderate amounts of alcohol (see below).

So that's it in a nutshell: more fruits and veggies, more fish, more beans and legumes, more whole grains, more nuts and seeds, more berries, more cheese, more olive oil, and more dark chocolate for desert. What could be more delicious, especially if you complement it all with moderate amounts of good red wine?

That said, many other specific foods and beverages are commonly promoted by health-food-nuts for their supposedly amazing health effects, such as brown rice, garlic, green tea, herbal tea, brewer's yeast, kelp, and soy products of all sorts. If you enjoy a kelp and nettle stew, followed by a soy burger, tofu desert, herbal tea, and a carob bar for desert, hey, all power to you because there's nothing wrong with ingesting more of those (although please don't invite me for dinner; I have other plans that night). It's just that there's nothing magical about any of them, no, not even soy. For example, one study on Hawaiian men found that those who ate the most soy ended up with the highest rate and most severe cases of Alzheimer's disease, "soybering" news indeed.

Finally, here are a couple of other healthy eating guidelines you may consider:

- Shop for your fresh produce as often as you can take the time. Fresh produce is not only healthier for you, shopping for food can be an easy and social form of exercise if you walk to the store and talk to the clerks.
- Read labels. I guarantee you will buy different brands of some products (say,

peanut butter) if you read what's in the brand you usually buy (salt, sugar, oils that are unpronounceable) versus what's in the healthier kinds.

- If you can afford it, buy organic, not because it's healthier (although it might be) but because an organic tomato tastes like a tomato should taste while a regular supermarket tomato tastes like a red baseball.
- Never ask for seconds. I know and you know, chances are that you took more than enough the first time around.
- Never skip meals. This is a no-brainer because you will just end up eating too much of the wrong things at the next meal.

Water

Water is so "in" these days that there are more brands of designer water than designer shoes. At least, that's the way it seems to the typical guy who can't tell a Blahnik from a blintz.

Everyone is drinking bottled water these days, even my mom, who decided that the only reason she couldn't keep up to the "old" people in her workout class (she's over eighty, they're over eighty-five, so they're really old) is that they had water bottles and she didn't. So I got her a water bottle and she claims to have made amazing strides as a consequence.

But how much water do you really need? And what kind of water should it be?

As I argued for years, studies have now revealed that you need a whole lot less water than most water enthusiasts push, and certainly less than most of you are drinking. In fact, experts are now so concerned about "over-hydration," which can dilute your blood and lead to very serious consequences (a runner in the 2002 Boston Marathon died as a result of over-hydration), that they have stated that, with certain exceptions such as working out in very hot circumstances, the best guide to determining your water needs is to drink only when thirsty and just enough to slake your thirst. That applies to exercisers and nonexercisers alike. In other words, no magic one-size-fits-all formula of eight glasses of water a day—drink when thirsty and no more.

What may surprise you even more is that to replace normal fluid needs, you don't have to focus all your attention on water because nearly any fluids will do (although I would certainly not advise that you try to meet all your fluid needs, as W.C. Fields reputedly tried doing, with scotch or rye; he hated water, he often said, because of what fish do in it). But coffee, for example, even though it's a diuretic, is OK as source of fluid intake, as are veggies, soups, fruits, and anything else that has lots of liquid in it, although clearly there are downsides to drinking too much soda pop or caffeinated beverages.

And as to the view of chauvinists that bottled water is so much more "pure" than other water sources, ha, ha, ha, because Dutch researchers determined that 40 per cent of bottled water samples contained enough bacteria and fungi to pose a potential threat to the well-being of people with immune deficiencies. Am I really laughing? No, just a little chortle is all.

Supplements, Minerals, Herbs

Let me first put my bias squarely on the table. Although I strongly believe in God (not sure of the gender, though), country (not saying which one), Manchester United (although now that they've been bought by an American developer who knows nothing about soccer, that may be on its way out; how can you root for a guy whose passion in life is floor plans?), the Habs (to my dying day, the team in my heart will be the Montreal Canadiens, my Rosebud, even in an eventually bankrupt and separated Quebec), roast chicken, and pike and carp only in gefilte fish (salmon in gefilte fish? Feh!), I don't believe in pushing supplements because I just can't see that in a world that has given us cashews and cantaloupe and cauliflower and Camembert that God or Darwin ever intended us to swallow a bunch of capsules every day instead of eating enough of the real stuff the capsules are intended to mimic. It's only our misplaced arrogance piled on top of our sloth that has allowed an industry of supplement pushers to convince us of the lifesaving properties of their overpriced potions. It's not that supplements are all harmful or useless. Many probably do some people some good, although surveys invariably find that those people who take supplements are usually the people who need them least, the dirty little secret the supplement industry always tries to hide when touting the claims made for supplements.

That said, most of the claims made on behalf of supplements are self-serving exaggerations meant to dull our much more urgent need to change our habits for the better. So, even if supplements do a bit of good, and that's a big if for most of them, taking vitamins E and C and beta-carotene and ginseng and lecithin and garlic capsules every day is never going to do you as much good as getting enough exercise and following a healthy, well-balanced diet that contains large dollops of all those vitamins and other good things.

Now that I have vented my spleen, I will say that as long as you have a healthy lifestyle, there are a couple of supplements that might be beneficial for you—so read on, brothers.

Vitamins

Most studies have shown that people who have higher blood levels of certain vitamins have better health outcomes than those who don't, which has led lots of people to advocate supplements to lower the risk of heart disease, nearly every cancer, dementia, degenerative conditions, neurological problems, inflammatory conditions, depression, asthma, and diabetes—not to mention that taking supplements can also lead to better immunity, better overall functioning, and improved ability to recite the Talmud.

I don't agree.

First, virtually every good study that has linked a health benefit to a higher blood level of some vitamin was done on people who ate the foods that led to those higher vitamin levels, not on people who took vitamin supplements.

Second, in nearly all such studies, it has been very difficult to tease out a single element (or often even several elements) that led to the better health outcomes. In other words, people who have higher vitamin levels often have lots of other reasons to end up with better health outcomes. They tend to be more educated, richer, have better jobs, eat much better diets, take more vacations, do more exercise, smoke less, perhaps even worry less (well, I would certainly worry less if I had more money, a better job, and took longer vacations), so how can a researcher easily extract one element—their subjects' vitamin C intake, say—and conclude that this is the sole reason those folks have lived longer or developed less disease?

Third, and this one gets far too little attention, in nature, vitamins and minerals are mixed in a proportion that manufacturers simply can't mimic, and it's very likely that it's that proportion that makes a huge difference in the effect we think we see from specific vitamins and minerals. "It's a team *heffort*," the humble Jean Beliveau always used to say after spearheading yet another Stanley Cup win by the Canadiens, and he was absolutely right. Similarly, in your body, vitamins and minerals put in a team effort, not a solo shot. God, after all, made a tomato with She-only-knows how many vitamins in delicate balance, and it's that combination, not simply its lycopene content, that gives the tomato its punch.

Finally, there's the very important fact that even vitamins are not without known risks (although in the doses most people take, vitamins are quite safe). For example, one very disputed study found that people who take high doses of vitamin E, strongly touted for its antioxidant properties, have a higher overall risk of dying than people who don't. Another study found that excess intake of vitamin C may worsen osteoarthritis, another concluded that people who take extra folic acid may develop dementia faster than people who don't, another that excess vitamin A leads to significantly higher risks of osteoporosis, and yet another that beta-carotene supplements led to quicker deaths in smokers who took the supplement than in smokers who chose not to take the supplement.

And don't be bought off with the argument that vitamins are "natural," with its implication that "natural" can't be nasty. Oh yes, it can. Arsenic is natural, after all. And so is melatonin, which is promoted for helping people sleep, but in animal studies melatonin has been found to shrink the gonads of Japanese quail. You don't really want to sleep better just to suffer shrinking testes, do you?

That said, there are possible exceptions to that general condemnation of supplement use. First, as stated earlier, in parts of North America, where the sun far too often don't shine even where it should shine, many of us are vitamin D deficient. And Vitamin D is important enough that I feel many of us could benefit by taking extra vitamin D (between 400 and 800 IU daily, perhaps as much as 1,000 IU).

Also, as we age, many of us have a diminishing capacity to absorb vitamin B_{12} (a recent Canadian study found that about one in five seniors is vitamin B_{12} deficient), and there doesn't seem to be any downside to taking extra vitamin B_{12} (vegans have to always take it in supplement form because vitamin B_{12} is only found naturally in animal products).

Finally, there's folic acid. While I, the jury, am still out on this one, folic acid may help lower the risk of heart disease (and other diseases linked to inflammation) in certain high-risk individuals (although a recent study determined that some people who take extra folic acid may progress to dementia faster than people who don't take it). Overall, I think this one may do more good than harm, especially if you have a high homocysteine level.

But that's it when it comes to my recommending supplements, except for some special circumstances and unusual situations (absorption problems, some chronic illnesses, and so on).

One final note: if, despite what I advise, you decide to take a particular vitamin because you think it will help you live longer, do not buy that bill of goods your local health food store might try to sell you about "natural-source" products. There is no proof that the much more expensive natural-source vitamins are any better than the synthetic vitamins, at least not better for you. They are certainly better for the bottom line of the people trying to sell you these overpriced panaceas.

Calcium

As I stated earlier, I don't believe strongly in a strict regimen of eating the recommended amount of calcium every day, which is 1,200 to 1,500 mg, but if you are going to go for it, try to do it through diet, especially dairy products (see above). If you can't stomach those, however, and if you don't particularly like salmon bones and whey—then by all means take calcium supplements, and no, it doesn't really matter whether it's calcium citrate or calcium carbonate—whichever one is easier on your pocketbook and your gut is fine by me.

DHEA (Dehydroepiandrosterone)

DHEA, a hormone produced in the adrenal glands and a precursor to both androgens and estrogen, is the current king of products for those people who get most of their health information on the Internet and who, like Trinity, believe in The One. And boy, do they believe. A partial list of what its proponents claim that DHEA can do for you includes postponing aging, lowering the risk of heart disease and cancer and inflammatory conditions, promoting sleep and weight loss, and on and on—everything, I think, except the ability to get you to appreciate gangsta rap, although I'll bet someone somewhere, probably in Philadelphia, is working on that one. As Keanu Reeves (The One) said so succinctly, "Wow."

So, yo, bro: are any of these claims valid? No one knows, because DHEA hasn't been studied in rigorous tests, and it probably never will be because it can't be patented. So it really doesn't pay the people who hype it to do the proper research since they can still make lots of money based on claims that will probably never be disproved. However, no one has ever shown that anyone taking DHEA has ever actually lived longer or better than people who don't take it, and besides, guys, some experts believe that DHEA might provoke a latent prostate cancer to grow more quickly (you can sit tight on that for a while).

Echinacea

An old joke:

Doctor: "Take this pill, Jack, and your cold will be gone in seven days."
Jack: "And if I do nothing, doc?"
Doc: "Then you'll be better in a week."

Echinacea, a herb, is widely promoted for boosting immunity, especially to prevent or treat the symptoms of a cold, so what I am about to say is unlikely to dissuade true believers from using echinacea the next time they come down with the sniffles. Nearly every good study has concluded that the study subjects who took placebo got over their colds in seven days, while the study subjects who took echinacea felt better in about a week. Case closed. By the way, want a better immunity booster for the next time you're down with a terminal cold, as all colds tend to be in men? Get ahold of Mrs. Hister and ask her for her garlic-laced chicken soup recipe. Be aware, though, that it starts with finding a kosher chicken. Good luck if you live in Flin Flon or Canmore.

Garlic

It is claimed that garlic can make arteries more flexible, that it can slow clotting, and that it lowers blood pressure and cholesterol levels. In addition, a U.S. study found that garlic prevented the growth of tumours in mice, although on the downside, garlic-eating mice lost all their non-Bulgarian friends. Hey, I love garlic and I promote it strongly (see chicken soup—above) but only because it tastes good, not because it might slightly lower your blood pressure.

Gingko Biloba

Every since a much-hyped study found that extracts of gingko biloba improved cognitive performance in some Alzheimer's patients, many people have been running out to buy some gingko—that is, when they can remember what to buy or why they went to the store in the first place. Bottom line: no real proof that gingko does much for the average yogi.

Selenium

A study in the *Journal of the American Medical Association* found that subjects who used 200 mg of selenium daily for four and a half years had their incidence of cancer reduced by 50 per cent, especially when it came to prostate cancer, colon cancer, and lung cancer. Selenium is being studied in several trials to see if it can indeed prevent cancer, so stay tuned, but don't buy into this yet.

Zinc

Zinc is promoted for its ability to boost immunity, especially in preventing colds and flus. A recent study also found that exercisers who ate a low-zinc diet experienced a significant drop in aerobic fitness as a consequence. Conversely, too much zinc can impair immunity and lower HDL cholesterol levels. Again, no real proof that zinc supplements matter. Instead, why not simply eat a diet with lots of zinc in it?

Finally, the million-dollar question: what do I, the conservative, skeptical author, take? Although when I first wrote *Midlife Man* I was taking supplements of vitamin E, folic acid, and calcium, I now eat a much better diet than I did back then, so I now take only extra vitamin D and vitamin B_{12}, but only when I remember (maybe I should start taking some gingko, too). And to be perfectly honest, I've never felt better, except for this persistent pain in my side, not to mention my memory lapses, my clotting abnormalities, and these bad moods that come over me all of a sudden. But hey, those are temporary, I'm sure.

Alcohol

"A glass of wine, taken with dinner/Leaves doctors' purses a little thinner." (Old English saying, not endorsed by the Canadian Medical Association.)

Most experts believe that a "moderate" intake of alcohol is good for most of us but an "excess" is bad. But how, exactly, does "moderate" differ from "excess"? I have always told my patients, as do all doctors, that "excess alcohol intake" is simply "anything more than I drink." A more objective answer is that moderate alcohol intake is one to two glasses of wine—or the equivalent amount of alcohol in other spirits—per day on most days. Not everyone agrees with this guideline, however.

On the one hand, a long-term study of physicians found that those male doctors who had two to four drinks a week had the lowest overall rate of death from all causes and that those who drank over one glass of alcohol a day had no increased life expectancy over teetotallers.

On the other hand, a Danish study found that three to five glasses of wine a day was correlated with the best health.

So which is it? Well, even if the Danes are right, I think that three to five glasses of wine a day is way too much to aim for, and certainly too much to recommend to the public, because we live in a society where most people believe that "if a little of something I like is good, a whole lot must be even better." So if we gave the green light to men to consume up to five glasses of wine or five beers a day guilt-free, many men would take that as tacit permission to drink even more (many already do), and they would consequently leave themselves open to all the problems excess alcohol intake leads to. I prefer to err on the side of caution and say that one to three glasses of wine a day is the maximum to consume regularly.

And remember it has to be drunk regularly, not in binges. So if you drink seven glasses of wine every Saturday and Sunday and you figure that that's the same as drinking two glasses of wine every night of the week (do the math; the answer is fourteen), it's not by a wide margin. Binge drinking is linked to far poorer health outcomes, and in fact, represents a serious health threat to our young folk, who seem to enjoy their alcohol in that fashion much more than we used to.

So, remember: Excess = bad. Moderate = good.

But that brings up the question of how good is "good"? To borrow from the evangelists: Good Is Great and it seems to be equally great nearly everywhere we look. Thus, in the U.S., a huge long-term study by researchers at the American Cancer Society determined that overall death rates were lowest among those who drank one alcoholic drink a day.

Not to be outdone by Americans, the Department of Public Health in Perth, Australia, found that the risk of mortality from all causes is about 15 per cent lower for people who drink some alcohol than for nondrinkers, a report that is well worth paying attention to, since Australians know more than most about alcohol. You could be stuck in the tiniest village in the remotest outcrop of an island on the coldest continent, but if you stumble into the moonshiner's kitchen, odds are that the first words you will hear will be the only other patron saying, "G'day, mate. Your shout?"

And then there are the Brits, who clearly like their pubs and love their ale. A study from England found that the "healthiest" group of Britons consisted of nonsmokers drinking 20 to 29 units of alcohol (one unit = one glass of wine, one small bottle or can of beer, or a one-ounce shot of hard liquor) each week. Ja, and Danish researchers concluded that drinking both red and white wine was associated with lower death rates overall in men between thirty and seventy.

Finally, of course, there's the French. Now the French clearly see the world unlike you and I do. I mean, they consider Jerry Lewis and Woody Allen icons, for Pete's sake, and they treat that buffoon, Gerard Depardieu, seriously. So it's certainly possible that the French might gather and interpret their statistics differently than we do. ("Eh, Jean, that Louis est mort, suddenly, you know, non pas from a bad heart, bien sur, but from eating too many snails and courgettes.") Nonetheless, most experts still agree that despite doing few of the things we think are essential to prevent heart disease, the French have overall lower levels of heart disease–related mortality than we do in North America—the famous French paradox. When I say that the French don't try to protect their hearts, here is what I mean. In North America, the experts tell us that if we want to protect our hearts, we have to avoid smoking, avoid high-fat foods, and do lots of aerobic exercise. And how do the French treat that advice? With a Gallic shrug, of course. As a frequent tourist to France, I can tell you that just by walking into a Paris bistro, restaurant, or pub, you will passively inhale one pack of Gauloises before you even hit your seat (next to a woman with a poodle named Chou-Chou on her lap, no doubt, who has his own place setting and growls if you look his way); that if you ask a Frenchman where you can find a low-fat meal, he will invariably smirk and point to England; and that the French do absolutely no aerobic exercise—after all, has anyone ever seen any Frenchman running? If you see a jogger in Paris, you can be sure he's from Louisville, not Lyons.

So what protects the French from an epidemic of heart disease? Most experts agree that it must be at least in part their alcohol intake, and to that end the French are great suppliers of statistics backing up this view. An excellent example is a report that followed 34,000 Frenchmen for fifteen years and found that moderate wine drinkers (which these French researchers defined as anyone drinking four—four—or fewer glasses of wine a day) had a 20 per cent lower risk of death from cancer than all other groups and a 20 to 30 per cent reduced risk of heart attack and brain hemorrhage, or stroke.

So moderate alcohol intake can help you live longer. Besides its beneficial effect on life expectancy, though, moderate alcohol intake may confer other health benefits as well:

- Regular intake of alcohol has been linked in many studies with lower risks of heart attack and stroke.
- Regular ingestion of alcohol has been linked with lower risks of Alzheimer's disease and other dementias.
- Wine may protect your stomach against infection with bacteria such as *Escherichia coli* (commonly known as *E. coli*), *Shigella*, or *Salmonella*. So on the next trip to Mexico, to hell with all the preventive antibiotics. Some Merlot by the minute, and hey, even if you get turista, you won't mind.
- Moderate alcohol consumption has also been associated with a decreased risk of infection with *Helicobacter pylori*, the bacteria that causes gastritis

and peptic ulcers, as well as lower rates of age-related macular degeneration (the leading cause of blindness in the elderly), and kidney stones.

- According to a study in the *Journal of Wine Research* (and I'm sure these guys have absolutely no bias), red wine can even help you recover from radiation poisoning. So the next time you're caught in a nuclear war, just get hold of a few bottles of plonk, and I'm sure all will end well.
- Finally, as Ogden Nash pointed out, "Candy,/Is dandy,/But Liquor,/Is quicker." A study from Finland concluded that two glasses of wine has an aphrodisiac effect on women, probably because alcohol raises testosterone levels in women. There was no equivalent effect on men, however, probably because men don't need wine to get more interested in sex.

All in all, then, moderate alcohol intake seems to be correlated not only with a longer life but also with a better quality of life. And the even better news for midlife guys is that, according to most estimates, the older you are, the greater the potential benefits, although I really doubt that means that a ninety-year-old has more to gain from regular tippling than a fifty-year-old does. What it does mean is that since the greatest benefit from regular alcohol intake seems to be its ability to lower the risk of heart attack, that benefit will clearly be greater for men who are at particularly high risk for this problem, so that middle-aged men and young seniors are likely to benefit much more from moderate alcohol intake than young men are.

But how, you may well wonder, does alcohol exert its positive effect? We don't know, but as usual, there are lots of theories:

- Moderate amounts of alcohol raise the levels of "good" cholesterol (HDL), perhaps more effectively than any other lifestyle adjustment.
- Alcohol may lower the levels of "bad" cholesterol (LDL) a bit, although it may have a slightly deleterious effect on blood levels of triglycerides.
- Alcohol may slow clotting of the blood.
- Some substances in alcohol have powerful antioxidant effects.
- The substance in red wine known as resveratrol may have an estrogenlike protective effect on tissues such as the heart and the brain (which is why, I suppose, whenever I drink a glass of wine, I get the urge to phone my sister, and I don't even have a sister).
- Alcohol lowers anxiety and stress levels. (I am certain that this is what exerts at least some of alcohol's positive effects. After all, drink a couple of glasses of wine and even your teenagers seem manageable.)

The most likely explanation, however, is some combination of all of the above.

But what about—the teetotallers are no doubt bursting to shout—alcohol's negative health effects, especially those on the brain? After all, alcohol is a powerful toxin and even a small amount of alcohol is bound to kill some brain cells.

Not in Scandinavia. According to a study from Denmark in which the brains of alcoholics were analyzed (at autopsy, I hope; I mean even in laid-back Denmark I'm sure they couldn't get away with doing it the other way) and compared with the brains of nondrinkers, there was no detectable difference between the two groups in number of neurons in the neocortex, the part of the brain associated with higher brain functions such as remembering where to find the Little Mermaid. There is one teeny caveat to all this, however, because when compared with teetotallers' brains, drinkers' brains were "shrunken" in other areas, such as those involved in sexual response, anger, fight-or-flight, and fear, a finding that could go a long way in explaining why men who drink a lot are always ready to challenge all comers that theirs is bigger than yours.

Alcohol doesn't seem to hurt Australian brains, either. A study of Australian veterans found that long-term moderate use of alcohol did not impair cognitive functions, although I am amazed that they were able to find Aussie soldiers who drank only moderately.

So moderate intake of alcohol doesn't kill brain cells or negatively affect cognitive functioning. In fact, it's probably quite the opposite in that many studies have linked moderate levels of alcohol intake to lower risks of dementia and better results in many cognitive areas in old age. Hey, I'll drink to that.

And it's the same for all other tissues, too: drinking moderate amounts of alcohol on a regular basis seems to exert no negative effects on—and may even protect—bones, muscles, connective tissue, and organs.

As for which type of alcohol is best, most studies claim to find only slight differences between equivalent amounts of wine and beer and to a lesser extent, hard liquor. As a committed wine drinker and an equally committed beer hater, however, I have to say that a snappy Shiraz (Merlot is sooo yesterday!) will clearly beat a bottled Bud every time. Thus, I prefer studies such as the one from Denmark I cited earlier, in which beer drinkers were not nearly as likely to benefit from their alcohol intake as were the winers like me, or a study from the University of North Carolina that found that drink for drink, beer guzzlers and hard-liquor drinkers were three times as likely to have a higher waist-to-hip ratio than wine drinkers. Since a high waist-to-hip ratio is correlated with higher rates of cardiac disease, winers' lower waist-to-hip ratio may help explain why they are better off than those big-butted, fat-waisted, couthless, smelly beer guzzlers.

No discussion of alcohol is complete, however, without also mentioning the very significant downside of excess alcohol. Do not be seduced by the glowing reports of alcohol's benefits: 10 to 20 per cent of the population cannot handle alcohol at all, and if you're one of those people, stay away from this (for you) very dangerous substance. Alcoholics are much more likely to suffer the negative consequences of alcohol well before the positive ones kick in.

Excess alcohol intake is related to a higher level of:

- heart attacks and strokes
- several cancers
- cirrhosis and liver cancer
- high blood pressure
- impotence
- neurological disorders
- dementia and other disorders of brain deterioration
- depression
- pneumonia
- kidney disease
- diabetes

Drinking too much is also linked to many other physical and psychological problems, including:

- impaired judgment
- poorer ability to cope
- accelerated aging
- impaired sleep
- poor weight control
- abdominal obesity
- depression and chronic anxiety
- much higher rates of death from suicide and accidents

Remember, too, that alcohol interacts with many medications, and it may be especially dangerous when you are also taking analgesics such as ASA, acetaminophen, and other over-the-counter painkillers. This potentially lethal combo has been linked to a higher risk of liver damage, bleeding from the stomach, and sudden death.

There's also this terribly important caveat: not only does excess alcohol intake often ruin the life of the drinker, it often ruins the lives of his or her family members as well. If you are drinking too much—and there are all sorts of self-administered tests and quizzes available on the Internet and from drug-and-alcohol agencies to help you determine if you have a problem with alcohol—then for your own sake as well as that of your family, friends, co-workers, and potential victims, seek some professional help. But seek it from a professional who knows what he or she is doing. Your old family doctor may not, I'm afraid, be the best person to help you unless your doctor is prepared to be very honest and harsh and is also willing and able to take the considerable amount of time needed to deal with you and your games.

Finally, if you don't already drink, there is absolutely no evidence that you should suddenly start drinking as soon as you finish this chapter (or sooner). Not only do teetotallers do pretty well in many studies, but there is also no proof that suddenly starting to drink alcohol in your middle years after a lifetime of abstention is going to help you live longer and better, although it will probably permit you to have more fun.

Having said all that, one last word: l'chaim!

Caffeine

Some sour souls have become captive to a hatred of caffeine that defies rational explanation, and now that the war on tobacco is nearly won, I am sure these zealots will turn their guns on caffeine so that we will soon, I fear, be witness to all sorts of restrictive anti-coffee laws, such as not being allowed to drink coffee in public buildings or restaurants except in special decaf sections, or even in planes ("this airplane is equipped with the latest coffee detectors in the washrooms, and anyone found drinking coffee will be thrown out in midflight"), all of which will no doubt be preceded by studies showing the terrible consequences of secondhand coffee intake. "Our study found that 80 per cent of mellow people sitting next to someone drinking a double cappuccino report becoming jumpy."

It is these coffee haters, I'm sure, who are behind all those studies that have claimed that caffeine is responsible for the following deleterious health effects:

- elevated cholesterol levels
- increased risk of heart attack
- increased risk of cancer of the pancreas
- osteoporosis

- a rise in blood pressure
- all sorts of mental, psychological, and physiological impairments, including decreased ability to think and concentrate as well as poorer performance on many tasks

To the chagrin of the coffee haters, however, nearly all these findings have been flushed away in subsequent followup studies, which have determined that moderate amounts of coffee are not associated with increased risks of osteoporosis, heart attack, or cancer, nor does coffee impair performance of any sort.

Why these differences in findings? Three main reasons. First, coffee is much more than a simple caffeine drip. Thus, coffee also contains potassium and magnesium and other elements, all of which more than likely balance out the potentially negative consequences of taking in caffeine. Second, most people who drink coffee regularly seem to quickly adjust to its effects—spike in heart rate, spike in blood pressure, a "buzz," and so on—and those effects soon evaporate in regular coffee drinkers. It's very hard, then, to tease out the role that this "accommodation" plays in many test subjects when studies are done on the effects of coffee. Third, the effects of coffee can vary significantly according to the manner in which the coffee is prepared.

Bottom line: if you are a healthy person, coffee in moderate amounts is not bad for you, and even if you're not healthy, it's unlikely that moderate amounts of coffee will do you harm. What may be even more disheartening to anti-coffee nuts, however, is that if you are not already jiving with java, perhaps you should be. Here are some of the potential benefits of coffee:

- A study has linked regular coffee intake with lower risks of at least two cancers: liver cancer and colon cancer, perhaps because the bowel, like a commuter on his twice-daily cross-town commute, much prefers a rapid transit time.
- Regular coffee drinkers (guilty!) have significantly lower risks of developing Type II diabetes.
- An excellent way for long-distance travellers to ease their jet lag is to force themselves to wake up at the appropriate hour in their new time zone and drink a couple of strong cuppas.
- Caffeine stimulates the central nervous system, producing a heightened sense of alertness, faster thinking, and an increased ability to pay attention (in between extra visits to the washroom, of course) while also minimizing fatigue.

- Caffeine dilates some arteries—although I would still recommend that you take an ASA instead of making a quick visit to a Starbucks at the first sign of a heart attack.
- Caffeine constricts arteries to the head, meaning that caffeine is useful as a headache remedy.
- According to Swiss researchers, coffee can neutralize cancer-causing chemicals in well-done meat.
- British researchers have found that drinking coffee can counter the effects of having a cold (a double cap sure beats two echinacea caps, if you ask me).
- Caffeine drinkers are less prone to depression and suicide, in part, I suppose because coffee drinkers are too hyper to kill themselves but probably also because coffee has a positive effect on brain chemicals such as serotonin.

Reluctantly, I must admit that coffee does have some downsides (which are certainly more of a problem in high-risk individuals):

- temporary small spikes in blood pressure
- a possible small rise in homocysteine levels
- caffeine withdrawal effects that can usually lead to headaches and lethargy (and are the reason that some people who drown themselves in coffee during the week but who swear off coffee on weekends to "relax" often spend the weekend making the rest of us feel more tense)
- interference with sleep, an effect that can apparently last up to twelve hours after the coffee is imbibed (so if you are having trouble sleeping, try to cut out that later afternoon coffee break to see if it helps)
- increased symptoms of gastroesophageal reflux disease (although interestingly, several studies have shown that this is an individualized effect—that is, many people can drink coffee without getting worse reflux)

Happily, though, even these seemingly intrusive negative effects can have an unintended positive consequence, to wit, at least one study has shown that seniors who drink coffee at night have more sex than seniors who don't drink coffee. Well, if you're going to be up late at night, how much Leno or Letterman can you watch anyway?

Finally, if you haven't yet learned to love coffee by the time you're fifty, I don't suppose that you ought to start drinking it now, even if it is bloody time you stopped being so damn mellow and self-congratulatory. Sorry about that. A little caffeine jumpiness there, I'm afraid.

{7}

PLAN B: THE HARDER WORK INVOLVED IN BECOMING HEALTHY

• • •

The wise for cure on exercise depend.

JOHN DRYDEN

Early to rise and early to bed makes a male healthy and wealthy and dead.

JAMES THURBER, "The Shrike and the Chipmunks," *Fables for Our Time*

OK, guys. I hope you've rested and recovered from reading that last chapter and that you're ready to plow on because I have some bad news for you. Chapter 6 was what I consider to be the easy stuff on how to stay healthy. After all, anyone can change his or her diet a bit, especially if it doesn't involve eating tofu, and most of you will also have very little trouble, I'm sure, drinking a few more cappuccinos and an extra glass or two of wine. But the sad fact is that even if you make all the changes I recommend in Chapter 6, that will still not be enough to live longer and better.

I know most of you don't want to hear this but it takes more than just changing what and how you chew or swallow to maximize your chances of being healthy when you hit your older years. It actually takes some effort. You can't get very healthy, I'm afraid, by just sitting on the couch or at the dining room table. And that's what this chapter is about—some of the harder work involved in improving your lifestyle. You must start to pay more attention to your weight and your sleeping habits, and most important, you must become more active.

"But why now?" you may well whine to your mate when she reads you this bit. "Why is Hister bugging me to become more active at this time in my life? Why not wait till I'm just a bit older, like seventy-eight, perhaps, before I start trying to stop the clock?" The answer to that is simple: although it's never too late to start living a healthier life, it's best by far to make healthy changes to your lifestyle in midlife. The Honolulu Heart Program, for example, has concluded that you get a much, much bigger bang for your buck if you make the appropriate lifestyle adjustments in midlife than if you wait a few years.

And lest you forget, midlife is where you is right now.

Weight Control

We who live in the developed nations are avoiring too much dupois, and we're padding that dupois with unseemly alacrity. Surveys reveal that more than two-thirds of American adults are overweight (BMI over 25—see below) and that about half are obese (BMI over 30), and those numbers are increasing every year! As usual, the Americans are out in front of the rest of us on this one, but the sad fact is that every developed nation is heading for a mountain of trouble from the legions of bowling-ball-shaped baby boomers plodding and shuffling into their dotage. In fact, one British study estimates that within five years, three out of four British guys are going to be overweight.

But how, you may wonder as you try to catch a glimpse of your toes this evening and consider whether it's worth reading on, are you supposed to figure out if you've even got a problem with weight? The experts always talk about BMI, or body mass index, a number derived by dividing your body weight in kilograms by your height in metres squared. Anything over 25 is potential trouble country, they say, and over 30 means that you should be reluctant to take your shirt off in public. How important is BMI? A study found that for every 1 per cent increase in BMI above the healthy lower range, there was a corresponding increase of 10 per cent mortality from all causes in young and middle-aged men.

BMI has its drawbacks as a universal standard of obesity, however, since it doesn't account for 1) where you store your weight (weight stored around the middle, for example, is much worse for you than weight stored on your head, or more likely, on your hips), and 2) how much of your weight is composed of muscle, which weighs more than fat (Lance Armstrong, for example, probably has a higher BMI than you do, but you know, I wouldn't worry too much about Lance if I were you).

Perhaps, then, an easier way to gauge your fat content (which is really all we're after here) is to simply measure your waist circumference with a tape that you can circle around your middle (yes, around the fattest point). If it's over thirty-four inches, you're probably entering trouble country (unless, of course, you're a lot like Lance). Still another way is to just look in the mirror. If the guy you see staring back at you looks much more like Jackie Gleason than like Jackie Chan—then it's time to shed a few pounds. By the way, a word of warning: don't lie to yourself. Use the tape measure, because studies show that when people merely estimate their girth or weight without direct measurement, they tend to drastically underestimate.

Why is excess weight bad for you? Because it can kill you. A study that looked at Harvard alumni for over thirty years, for example, found a "straight-line" relationship between weight and mortality; men who weighed 20 per cent less than the average for their height had the lowest mortality rate, whereas men who were obese had the highest mortality rate. I must point out, however, that this claim that being overweight or obese kills hundreds of thousands of us a year has recently been called into question by a much-cheered study from the Centers for Disease Control in the U.S. that concluded that the death rate from obesity is far lower than most experts have claimed. In fact, these researchers claim that those who are slightly overweight are less likely to die than those who have a "normal" weight. Needless to say, this study has raised a real fuss among the medical number-crunchers, and as I write this, the stats are hitting the fan, big-time, with most experts condemning this ballyhooed conclusion, and I must say I am in the latter camp. Thus, I choose to stick with the "obesity kills" crowd, because I just can't imagine that being fat and lazy is what God planned for our eventual best ends.

But how, you may also be wondering, can excess weight possibly kill someone? Most important, through its deleterious effect on the heart and cardiovascular system. Several studies, including the fifty-year-long Framingham study, have revealed that obese people end up with:

- higher blood pressure
- higher levels of inflammation
- higher levels of injury to cardiac arteries
- larger hearts
- thicker walls in the pumping chambers of the heart

All of the above are linked to an increased risk of premature heart disease and death. Even a small increase in weight can raise your risk of having a heart attack when you have no other risk factors for coronary heart disease. The Nurses' Health Study, for example, found that a weight gain of as little as twenty-two pounds over what a woman weighed at age eighteen leads to an increased risk of death in midlife. Now I know that most guys reading this will immediately say, "Hey! I don't ever plan on becoming a fat nurse, so who cares?" But that would be a very foolish thing to say, guys, because not only do you not know what the future holds—after all, as part of a midlife crisis you may very well go back to school and become a nurse, and you might even change your mind about gender surgery. I see no reason to believe that similar results would not apply to non-nursing men as well.

Heart disease aside, excess weight is correlated with a higher risk of many other diseases. In fact, according to a fascinating survey of 73,000 people, being overweight resulted in higher risk of forty-one separate health conditions and problems, including most importantly:

- Type II diabetes
- high blood pressure
- osteoarthritis
- gallstones
- strokes
- blood clots
- several types of cancer, including colon cancer, esophageal cancer, kidney cancer, and liver cancer
- depression
- dementia
- premature and accelerated aging (the cells of middle-aged obese people have been found to be eight to ten years older than the cells of people at normal weight)

There are a couple of caveats, however. First, clearly, many very heavy people live to a ripe old age. How do they do it? Well, most of them are very fortunate souls, blessed with great genes and even better luck.

But that's not the only factor that may play a role. Fitness counts for a lot, too, probably even more than weight. Some of you may find this hard to imagine, but you can be fat and fit at the same time, and people who are fit and fat do all right. In fact, statistics from the Cooper Institute for Aerobics Research show that overweight men who are fit have a lower risk of dying from heart attack than thin men who are not fit. The good news is, then, that if you are fit, living within the vicinity of your ideal weight is probably good enough, and even living within a commuting suburb of the ideal is probably OK, too. But you have to be fit!

Equally important, it's not only how much you weigh but where you carry those pounds that's crucial in determining many of the health risks associated with excess weight. Thus, someone who carries excess weight around the middle (in the classic apple shape) rather than on the hips (in the classic pear shape) is in a heap more trouble than his Bartlettian bro. Weight around the middle is linked to a much higher risk of insulin resistance, which is in turn related to a much higher risk of heart disease, stroke, and the whole enchilada that comes with Type II diabetes. Now clearly, some of the weight we carry and where we carry it is beyond our control, a product of our genes. Thus, a study from Toronto showed that although your lifestyle may determine that you end up looking like a Macintosh apple, your genes might determine whether you become a big Mac or a small Mac, and those of us who are small Macs are less likely to develop obesity-related problems than are our Fuji-wannabe brothers. Overall, another study estimated that from 20 to 40 per cent of obesity is determined by your genes. But the other side of that fat coin is that 60 to 80 per cent of your excess weight is probably under your control, and it's those extra pounds that you want to attack.

So what should you do? Well, the bottom line, especially as it sags nearer and nearer to the ground, is this: if you are too fat for your height, there are really only two ways to attack this unfair problem. One is to grow taller. The other is to try to lose weight.

And there are also only two ways to lose weight: Do more. Eat less. Thank you very much, and you can mail the Nobel Prize to my home because I don't really ever want to visit Stockholm. Too many dour and smug professors in too many Volvos and Saabs.

Why do more? Because (except for some exceptional specimens) the more you do, the lighter you should get, assuming, of course, you don't compensate for the extra work by eating more. But also, the more you work, the more fit you will get, and in the end, I think that being fit is more important than weighing less.

Doing more involves a twofold strategy: becoming more active in your daily routine and starting to do regular exercise. As to which exercise is best, any exercise that raises caloric output without at the same time increasing the urge to eat more will help (see the next section, on exercise).

You have to learn to eat less, too. That one is clearly not easy, as the multibillion-dollar weight-loss industry can attest. Alas, despite scientists' frantic push to satisfy western society's most urgent need—to find a tiny pill that taken once a day, or even better, once a month, would allow us to have our cake and eat it too (and most of us would eat the entire cake if we could)—for now, there is no such pill available, although that may change soon when rimonabant comes along (not only for weight loss but also as a stop-smoking aid—Jackpot City for its makers). Rimonabant has been hyped beyond belief in prerelease studies, with some reports indicating that the 5 to 10 per cent of body weight lost on this pill could be kept off for up to two years, which is very impressive. Before you sell the family jewels to buy as many rimonabant shares as you can get ahold of, though, please remember fen-phen and all the other pretty pills that promised the same thing. Every weight-loss pill that has come along has resulted in rare but potential health risks that far outweighed the potential benefits for anyone not seriously overweight, and I, the jury, will be out on rimonabant until it's been on the market for at least five years, and I advise you to do the same. So for now, demonstrating willpower and following a healthy diet remain the best strategies to lose weight. Which diet? you ask. It really doesn't matter. So long as you keep a lid on your portion size and the number of portions you help yourself to (a calorie is just a calorie, après tout), every diet is equally effective in the short term. So just pick a diet you think might work and go for it, although there are restrictions to some diets that you should be aware of. For example, if you have gout, don't go on a high-protein diet. Just remember what your grade four teacher said, and do your homework first.

Bottom line: there is absolutely no proof that any diet—from Pritikin to Scarsdale to Dean Ornish to The Zone to Atkins to South Beach to Styrofoam chips and salsa—has any better track record than another when it comes to helping you stick with it or helping you keep the excess weight off.

Also, it might pay you to follow a few other strategies at the same time as dieting. A long-term study of people who lost at least thirty pounds and kept it off for a few years found that they all:

- ate breakfast every day (easy)
- weighed themselves often (really easy)
- exercised at least one hour a day most days of the week (not so easy)

Other strategies that have come out of the plethora of studies done on dieters include:

- eating as many meals as possible as a family: family meals tend to be much healthier than meals eaten solo in every way, including portion size
- eating fewer foods: as anyone who loves his buffet meals (guilty!) will tell you, the more choices you have, the more food you will pack away (you might even take a leaf from my mom's book and for dinner serve one portion of

boiled meat, one portion of boiled potato, and one portion of wilted salad—I guarantee you will lose weight on that diet)
- adding lots of water dense foods such as salads to your meals: an interesting study from Pennsylvania State University found that dieters who focused on adding water-dense foods (mostly fruits and veggies) to their meals ate far fewer calories as a consequence (apparently, you tend to eat the same volume of food no matter what, so why not fool your stomach with high-volume, lower-calorie choices?)

One thing I would not do is depend on low-fat or low-cal drinks and sodas. Why? Because there really is no substitute for eating less. In the end, all successful diets work because of one factor, and one factor only: they lessen your calorie intake. Period. And anything that deflects you from eating less is, I think, only setting you up to fail at weight loss. As evidence, I'll cite an interesting but not surprising study that found that the more diet soda people drank, the more weight they gained. Specifically, for every can or bottle of diet soda consumed every day, there was a corresponding 41 per cent increase in the risk of being overweight. It's not that the diet soda leads to weight gain (although that is possible). Rather, it's that when people start to focus on diet products to lose weight, they stop focusing on the much more important issue of calorie control. As proof, I offer myself as Exhibit A: every time I pig out on Chinese food, I assuage my conscience by ordering a diet Coke.

I also encourage you to never stop trying to lose weight, if that is your goal. Don't be afraid to try dieting from time to time, and if you relapse, take time out and give it a go again when you're ready. You can succeed. Lots of people have. Yo-yo dieting is unlikely to be bad for your health, and losing some weight even temporarily is probably better for you than just accepting the excess poundage and doing nothing about it.

It can be done. It just takes effort, persistence, discipline, and patience.

Finally, I am going to end this section with a bit of a downer, I'm afraid. Even if you work hard at trying to lose weight, it may still not be enough. According to a very depressing study, even men who run a fair amount still gain weight and spread around the middle as they hit middle age, which means that as you grow older, you will have to continue to increase the amount of exercise you do just to stay at the same weight. Sorry to end it like this, but at least you can go have a glass of wine now to cheer yourself up. Have to work that wine off later, though.

Exercise for the Body

Too many of us are too sedentary. A U.S. survey found that by age sixty-five, the average North American will have spent the equivalent of nine years in front of the tube, and that survey was done even before *Seinfeld* reruns went into syndication. So imagine how bad it is now.

In Canada, a report prepared for the Heart and Stroke Foundation found that 35 per cent of Canadians are "essentially inactive," meaning that inactivity has now officially replaced constitution-kvetching as Canada's national sport. What's worse, the more people move to the suburbs, the more sedentary they tend to become, so the continuing suburbanization of North America is only going to make matters worse.

But why, many of you flat on your backs while reading this might want to know, should you even bother exercising? What benefits can regular exercise offer you? For one thing, it extends life, which is not a bad thing for most of us. In fact, according to many experts, slothfulness is more of a risk for premature death than being obese. Want proof? One large study of middle-aged guys that lasted six years found that their exercise capacity on a treadmill was the best predictor (better than cholesterol levels or blood pressure or glucose levels) of which guys would survive and which ones they had to honour with a celebration of their lives. So just how far can *you* run without getting breathless?

Regular exercise also lowers the risk of developing nearly every disease and condition you can think of, including the keys ones:

- heart disease
- stroke
- several cancers
- osteoporosis
- Type II diabetes
- Parkinson's disease
- disability of daily living (meaning that the more fit you are, the fewer physical limitations in daily living you end up with as you age)

Exercise also leads to:

- better weight control
- loss of fat, especially abdominal fat
- replacement of fat with muscle
- better immune system functioning

- less pain and inflammation
- lower blood pressure
- higher levels of HDL cholesterol (even in the absence of weight loss, please note!) and lower levels of LDL cholesterol
- improved fat distribution
- more flexible blood vessels
- improved action of the heart
- lower risk of neurological diseases
- better quality of sleep
- less deterioration in hearing and sight
- much less ED
- fewer days off work

Perhaps most important for baby boomers terrified of developing Alzheimer's disease, exercise is particularly beneficial for the brain. Studies have shown that regular exercise leads to:

- better memory
- better moods
- better control of depression
- lower levels of stress
- lower risk of dementia
- better scores on cognitive tests
- increased creativity
- enhanced alertness (a study from Manchester University concluded that a group of "super-fit" seventy-year-olds was just as alert as a group twenty years their junior, although given the level of alertness of the average fifty-year-old, sleep-deprived adult, I'm not sure that's such a great claim to make)

Exercise may even help the brain repair itself. Dr. Rodney Swain from the University of Wisconsin in Milwaukee found that rats that enjoyed running (although to be honest, I still can't picture a jogging rat—it's the tiny spandex shorts I have the toughest time with) grew new blood vessels in the brain within three days of starting to run.

Finally, for me, the biggest benefit of doing a lot of exercise is that I get to eat more without regaining the weight I took off six years ago.

"Sure, sure, that's all great," many men reading this are probably saying. "But so far, Art, you haven't said anything about what effect exercise has on sex." Well, it certainly can't hurt and it might even help—a lot. One researcher has claimed that exercise is a "sure fire way to reawaken your sexual spirit," and you know, until I read that, I had absolutely no inkling that I even had a sexual spirit, something that made me wish that I had spent more time on my spiritual nature in my younger years.

So now that I've convinced you of the need to do more exercise, we need to establish how much exercise you should do. Here, I'm afraid, the jury is still out and farting around. You see, in an attempt to encourage more people to do more, or even to do anything, many health experts have abandoned their decades-long exhortation to do vigorous exercise many days a week, and they are now claiming that as little as thirty minutes of extra work, involving as little activity as puttering around the garden, even taken in ten-minute hits three times a day, is enough: "exercise lite" to accompany your cholesterol-free eggs and fat-free mayonnaise.

But is exercise lite really good enough? It all depends on what you want out of your exercise regimen. Besides the feel-good aspect of doing exercise, there are really only three significant benefits to be gained from exercise:

- weight loss and weight control
- an improved aerobic fitness level
- a lower risk of chronic diseases associated with a sit-on-your-ass lifestyle

Each of these probably requires a different level and intensity of exercise.

To lose weight and to keep it off, exercise lite is rarely enough. Why? Because a calorie is a calorie, so the more calories you burn through effort, the more weight you will lose, although sadly, some people can't lose weight no matter how much they exercise. But before you immediately look at your wife and say, "Hey, hon, that's me to a tee and that's why I don't do more," please note that this applies to only a very small minority of people. Trust me on this. You—yes, you—don't belong to that group. Keep after him, hon.

If, however, you're satisfied with your weight and you merely want to do enough exercise to stave off illness, exercise lite may be enough, although there is clearly still lots of dispute about this. So, on the one hand, a study of Harvard alumni found that vigorous exercise (a minimum of 2,000 or more calories expended per week) was correlated with better health, while non-vigorous exercise didn't do much for the best and brightest and most often quoted. On the ubiquitous other hand, a study from the Cooper Institute for Aerobics Research found a 15 per cent decline in mortality going from moderate fitness to high fitness but a 40 per cent lower mortality when going from no fitness to any fitness at all. In other words, a little pain, lots of gain.

I'm with the Cooper guys on this one. If all you want to do is prevent diabetes and heart disease and all those other conditions we mentioned earlier, thirty minutes of aerobic activity most days of the week (brisk walking is perfect, but make it brisk) is probably enough.

Finally, if you want to achieve a really good fitness level, the harder you exercise, the more fit you will become, although you should keep in mind, as I am forced to do every time I tell my trainer (or my wife) that I'm satisfied with my level of fitness, that this may be a Sisyphean task because according to the fitness nuts out there (sorry, dear) you can never really be fit enough. "You only did twenty reps? What's wrong with you? I can do thirty. And so can your mother." And so it starts again.

Now what about exercise equipment? Here I am a real conservative. I believe that the late Dr. George Sheehan, the original guru of the fitness movement in North America, had it right when he said, "All you need to get fit is to live in a two-story house, and have a poor memory." You don't need fancy step machines and treadmills to become fit. Even if you buy one of those overpriced gadgets, chances are you won't be using it after a few weeks anyway. I once saw a study claiming that most exercise bikes in the home are now used as clotheshorses, leading some wag to speculate that a smart company should market an exercise bike with the clothes hangers already attached.

That said, one bit of exercise equipment you should never skimp on, especially if you choose to run or walk, is your shoes and socks. Hey, your feet are precious, so do everything you can to minimize trauma to them. Spending a few extra dollars on a pair of runners that fit you better than the Wal-Mart bargain pair is going to be an investment you never regret (unlike the other great investment you made in something your barber guaranteed was bound to become the next *Harry Potter*).

Once you've decided to do more exercise, another big problem is what kind of aerobic exercise to pick. That one is actually easy. Walking every day is the best exercise regimen for most of you. Walking gets you outside, walking can be done anywhere, walking is cheap, walking is not swimming (I hate getting wet), walking is not linked to many injuries or hazards as long as you watch out for cars and dog poo, and walking can easily be done with a partner, adding a social benefit to the activity—but only if you like the partner. A partner has other benefits, too. Not only is exercise more pleasant when someone else is suffering along with you, but a partner will often motivate you when you don't have the oomph to get out that day. And it's unpleasant to let an expectant partner down too often.

If for some reason you can't walk—if you have severe arthritis of the hip or knee, for example, which makes if difficult to walk—then a good alternative is to buy yourself a stationary bike. Just put it in front of the tube and peddle away. Or do aqua exercises, if, unlike me, you can stand getting wet.

So that's formal aerobic exercise. Just as important, though, you should also aim to increase your calorie expenditure in your normal day-to-day activity. And to illustrate just how important regular day-to-day activity is in maintaining good health, consider the Amish. Yes, the Amish.

Have you ever wondered why every Amish man looks like he's 108 years old but still vigorous enough to put up your barn? By himself? Go on, yes, you have, and the answer is simple: it's because they walk so much in their daily activities. How much do they walk? Well, someone had the bright idea of attaching a pedometer to some Amish folk, and what they discovered is that while you and I rarely get over 3,000 to 4,000 steps a day, Amish men walked—are you sitting down? I'll bet you are because you're not Amish—an average of 18,000 steps a day, which also allowed them to eat 3,600 calories a day without getting fat.

We're very un-Amish, I'm afraid, and it's costing us dearly. I can't believe, for example, the number of people who use an elevator to go up one flight of stairs, who never move their butts while on an escalator, or who get their wives to take out the garbage (well, it's only because unlike me, my wife never confuses the garden trash cans with the regular garbage cans). If you were simply to take the stairs each time instead of the elevator or walk to the store regularly instead of driving, you would probably improve your chances of living longer even more than you would by suddenly taking up jogging or power walking. (But do continue to have your kids or wife take out the garbage because taking out the garbage isn't likely to help you live longer.)

You might also, by the way, just try to fidget a lot more. According to a study from the Mayo Clinic, it's your "non-exercise activity thermogenesis" (NEAT) that most determines if you're fat or thin. NEAT includes all those small movements and activities we do all day long and that, according to this study, can add up to lots and lots of calorie expenditure and can also explain why some people who don't do much exercise are still so thin.

But that's not all. You must also bear in mind that aerobic exercise is only one of the four categories of exercise we should all be doing regularly. The others are resistance training (you and I call that doing weights), flexibility exercise, and balance retraining.

For me, this has meant a combination of core exercises, weight training, and yoga, which I'm pleased to say has dramatically improved my chronic low back pain.

Resistance training is very helpful in maintaining muscle mass as we age, and even more helpful in replacing fat with muscle, so resistance training is probably most important for people like me, who had little or no discernible muscle mass to begin with. It's also helpful in improving aerobic exercise capacity and helping with balance. As well, resistance training can help maintain bone mass, improve energy levels, prevent diabetes, and elevate mood. ("I did it. I did it. I lifted that four-pound weight.") Plus, it can make you look more buff.

This is one area of training, though, that you really should not do on your own until you have had some good sessions with a person who knows that they're doing and who can teach you the right way to do the lifts and reps and all the rest of it. Believe it or not, there is a right way to do a curl and a wrong way to do a curl, and if you do it the wrong way (as I always did when left on my own), you substantially raise the risk of injuring yourself. Not only that, studies have indicated that beginners who do resistance training on their own generally take it too easy on themselves, what my wife calls "cheating" when I do it, "being smart" when she does it.

You should also start doing flexibility exercise regularly because flexibility also plummets with age. Want to see how much? Just drop this book and try to pick it up. Without groaning and krechtzing and kvetching (krechtzing is the sound all old people make when straining to use even a single muscle group; kvetching is the sound of the complaints that ensue). That's how much. Thing is, though, it's easy to regain a lot of that lost flexibility. And this is not an idle claim on my part, because if I can do it, you can do it. You see, about six months ago, on the advice of my newly flexible son (the first Hister in history to ever do a plow), I started doing yoga twice a week, and I can now nearly touch my toes (yes, that's with nearly straight legs). And if you don't think that's much of an achievement, you should know that no Hister male since the seventeenth century (the earliest year for which we have records) has come within even a few inches of touching his toes (not that very many Hister men in the shtetls of Poland tried, of course, but they couldn't have even if they'd wanted to). I'm nearly there, however, and at the advanced age of fifty-nine.

And then there's balance. You'll want to check on this one, too. OK. Try balancing on one leg with your eyes closed, but make sure you are away from sharp objects. OK, never mind—try simply balancing on one leg with your eyes open. See what I mean? You never knew your balance had gone so much, did you? Well, balance retraining, too, should be worked on regularly as part of an overall fitness regimen because as we age, falling and shattering bones can have devastating consequences for our lives (see Chapter 5). The good news is that the exercises you need to do to retrain your proprioception skills are simple and can be learned easily off the Internet or from a fitness book. But the trick is to start doing them and then to keep doing them regularly.

So there you have the elements of a basic exercise program:

- aerobic exercise
- resistance training
- flexibility exercise
- balance retraining

However, since everyone has different needs, different interests, and different amounts of time to devote to this part of life, it's up to you to pick what you want and put it into a package that suits you best.

Having touted the praises of walking—either alone or with a partner—let me now make a few positive comments about fitness clubs and trainers. First, a trainer at a fitness club can provide you with the discipline to stick with exercising that you might not have on your own. This is really important for me. It's not that my trainer is such a great disciplinarian. It's just that I prepay for my classes and I'll be damned if I'm just going to let the money line his pockets without having him do somthing to earn it.

Also, a good trainer can help you do the exercises the way they're meant to be done. As I admitted earlier, I cheat a lot in my exercise routines. Hey! It's lots easier to do a full set of curls if you only lift the bars half-way. My trainer, however, never allows me to cheat (when he can spot my cheating, that is), and I get much more benefit out of my routine that way.

Also, having a trainer or joining a class means that there's always someone to talk to during your otherwise tedious workout. The disadvantage, of course, is that I am so fed up with hearing about the problems that a thirty-year-old unattached guy has that I'm seriously considering sending my trainer for some counselling.

Before closing this section, I must address the most important potential downside to exercise, namely that exercise can kill you. But before you jump up (well, get up slowly) to throw your new and still-unused runners in the recycling pile, bear in mind that you may hurt yourself with that sudden movement, and besides, although sudden intense activity can kill, the benefits of an exercise program are far greater than that tiny risk. Anyway, that risk can be minimized by participating in exercise on a regular basis.

As to concerns about exercise harming your tissues, if you pick an activity that doesn't involve undue pounding (walking rather than running, for example), exercise is very unlikely to have any harmful effects on any body tissues or parts such as your bones or your joints, although if you develop any pain that isn't going away with the old TLC, then don't just tough it out and say, "Art said this would be good for me"—but make sure to check it out.

One final word: the secret to doing exercise is simple. Just do it. Pick an activity you might like, check with your doctor to make sure there's no reason not to do it (that's mandatory for a previously sedentary middle-aged chap, whether you were a great high school athlete or not), and then just do it. If that activity doesn't work out after a few weeks, give it up and pick something else, and just do that one.

Ask any successful exerciser and he'll tell you the same story. Sure, there are tons of excuses he can use every day, but in the end, he puts them aside and just does it. And so can you. And once it's part of your routine, studies show you're going to miss it when you don't do it. I promise.

Exercise for the Mind

In addition to keeping your body in good shape, you should make sure to do the same with your mind. But is there really anything you can do to counter the ebbing tide of your cognitive functions, you ask, short of carrying around a twenty-four-hour-pager and wearing an "If found, please return to..." sign around your neck? To a certain extent, yes.

For a start, you can stay healthy. A study from Scotland found that Scots who remain healthy into old age also maintain their full youthful intellectual abilities, although I leave it to your imagination as to how they were able to determine the difference between a Scot with diminished intellectual functions and a "normal" one. Did the researchers give them some haggis or another oatmeal product to see what they did with it? What would the right answer be anyway?

Then you can work on your female side, since women are better than men at remembering lists and people's names. Try shopping and buying several pairs of shoes at once, for example. Or how about calling one of your mates to discuss, well, I'm not sure what they discuss so ask your spouse for ideas, but call often and for any reason. As well as working on your female side, you should:

- Get a good education. The higher your level of education, the better your memory and other cognitive abilities in old age.
- Keep your stress level down. Studies suggest that chronic stress leads to memory impairment.
- Keep your blood sugar as low as you can by maintaining a healthy weight and doing lots of exercise. Both obesity and diabetes have been linked to loss of brain tissue.
- If you're already drinking some wine regularly, keep it up because studies show that moderate levels of alcohol intake are linked to better memory and cognitive skills in old age. ("Now, where did I leave that bottle of wine? Oh yes, I remember.")
- Keep your blood pressure down. High blood pressure in middle age has been linked to impaired cognitive abilities in later life.
- Keep physically active. Several excellent studies show that regular exercise retards memory loss.
- Keep mentally active. The old adage applies to cognitive skills, too—the more you use it, the less you lose it—so much so that studies suggest that even playing cards and going to bingo seems to help maintain better memory in old age. Hey, you think it's easy to remember what goes under the B?

You might also try to prevent that brain burnout mentioned earlier (see Chapter 2). Specifically, Dr. Ruben Gur, professor of psychiatry at the University of Pennsylvania and a leading expert in this area, told the London *Times* that "men may need to relax their brain in the same way they relax their muscles," not as much of a leap as you may think for the many men whose brains are largely muscle tissue anyway.

But relaxing your brain does not mean not using it at all. What you want to aim for is to use different parts of your brain, to exercise different brain functions than you usually do because the more flexible your brain is and the more varied stimulation it ends up receiving, the more synapses you build up over the years and the less it seems to fade with time.

This advice holds true throughout life. Thus, a study of Swedish twins concluded that 38 per cent of our ability to acquire and process knowledge is a product of our environment, and that even older adults can still process new information and learn new skills. By the way, this figure also means, unfortunately, that our genes account for 62 per cent (100 less 38 equals 62, except if you're my ex-accountant, although maybe even he would come up with this answer now that he has been able to do some remedial math in prison) of our general cognitive skills in old age, and that is something we can't affect.

"Absolutely terrible news," screamed my son Tim when I gave him this information. "Don't be silly," I shot back with a snide look at my wife. "You're OK. After all, you got half your brains from me." "That's what he meant," she smirked.

As to more active treatment, it is likely we will soon have drugs to rejig the brain and its functions. Although scientists have always believed that after a brain cell dies it stays dead and can never be replaced, recent research has shown that the brain can regrow some cells. Thus, it is very likely that one day scientists will find drugs that can regrow some of those passed-away neurons. As well, several recent studies have looked at what the researchers call a "memory pill," and the results are beginning to look up. There will always, however, be some major problems associated with such drugs, because not only are you going to have to remember to take one in the first place, but you will also have to remember where you last left the pillbox.

Sleep

Sleep is like the federal budget: it's just too easy to run a deficit and pretend that you will pay it back one day.

We haven't always been that dumb, though. The feds used to balance their budgets, and we used to sleep when we were tired. One hundred years ago, the Better Sleep Council claims, the average North American slept 20 per cent longer than we do now. Adults in 1900, who did not have the allure of all-night, mind-blowing entertainment like *Seinfeld* reruns on for the twelfth time and infomercials starring Cher, slept about nine and a half hours a night. Today, 60 per cent of modern-day Americans get an average of less than seven hours of sleep. And that's a particular problem for midlife men because studies show that in men, the quality of sleep starts to deteriorate in early adulthood, or soon after the peak in our sexual functioning (I have still not warmed to that latter theory, by the way, because if that was truly my peak, well, I am not eager to see the depths of my valley). Anyway, from around the age of twenty-five or so onwards, researchers have determined that it becomes harder for men to fall asleep, to stay asleep, and to get as rested from sleep, so that any artificial interruption with sleep penalizes us aging guys even more heavily than it does, say, a seventeen-year-old.

Sleep deprivation exerts a heavy price, both in immediate and in long-term effects on our health and well-being. On an immediate level:

- Fatigue from lack of sleep is a major contributor to motor vehicle accidents. According to one study of subjects' reflexes, for example, even moderate levels of fatigue led to "impaired performance" comparable to the performance deficit seen at a blood alcohol concentration of .05 per cent, and the researchers weren't referring to the kind of performance deficit most men usually worry about either.
- Any interruption of the normal sleep schedule for only a few hours causes people to be moodier and more anxious.
- Sleep deprivation has a negative effect on higher brain functions and cognitive skills, with subsequent negative effects on motivation, perception, and performance.
- Even three hours of sleep deprivation can lower immunity by decreasing the number of circulating "natural killer cells," those mean little Oliver Stones that nab any predators that dare invade your body. The good news is that a good night's sleep quickly restores those cell levels to normal.
- Because memories and learning are consolidated during sleep, any new skills you acquire may not be so easily stored and recalled if that learning is followed by a poor night's sleep.

The long-term effects of poor sleep are harder to gauge, but several studies have linked chronic sleep abnormalities with greater disability and poorer health outcomes, even with reduced life expectancy. Also, some researchers have recently proposed that chronic lack of sleep is partly responsible for the huge increase in obesity among North Americans. The theory is that lack of sleep disturbs hormone systems, which leads to less satiation, increased hunger, and poorer insulin control, although on a more immediate level, the more you're awake, the more time you have to eat. My son loved this theory, by the way. "So I guess what they're saying, Dad, is that if I want to control my weight, I should sleep more, right? Thanks, I think I will," and he hung up the phone, no doubt to nap.

How much sleep do you need? Most people seem to require eight to eight and a half hours of good sleep per night, but many people do fine on only six or even fewer and other people need eleven hours. The only way to gauge this is to see how tired you are following a certain number of hours of sleep.

But the number of hours you sleep should never be the sole determinant in helping you figure out if you're sleeping enough. You must also get good quality sleep, and again, the best way to determine that is to note how rested you feel the next day. If you are full of vim and vinegar, then you probably slept well enough, even if it was only a few hours. If you are tired and falling asleep at your desk, then it's either time to get a new job or time to work on sleeping better—or both.

How can you maximize the quality of sleep?

Start with keeping to a regular sleep schedule. Getting married also helps, since surveys reveal that married people tend to sleep better (and the longer you are married, the more sleep you get; see Chapter 3 on monogamy and sexual frequency). Other sound sleep-stimulating strategies include getting rid of anything in the bedroom that might disturb your sleep, such as a TV or a flea-bitten early-rising mutt, not eating heavily before bedtime, and getting more exercise during the day, which has been shown in several studies to improve quality of sleep and ability to fall asleep. You should also avoid late-evening ingestion of any substance that can interfere with sleep, such as alcohol, coffee, and the many drugs that contain caffeine. For the older midlifers, remember that any liquids at all in the evening are likely to result in unwanted tromps to the toilet at three A.M.

You should also note that many medications are well known for interfering with sleep, including some kinds of:

- antihistamines (interestingly, lots of people use the older antihistamines as sleeping potions because of those drugs' well-known tendency to lead to drowsiness)
- high blood pressure medications
- hormones
- antidepressants
- asthma drugs

Clearly, if you have to take these drugs to control a condition, the benefits probably outweigh the risks, but discuss all that with your doctor.

But say you've done all the above and you're still not sleeping well. What should you do next? That's when most people turn to a variety of home remedies such as:

- warm baths
- siestas (which are promoted by some experts, derided by others)
- various relaxation techniques
- sex (but only if it relaxes you)
- herbal tea
- valerian
- warm milk (the world's favourite sleep potion)

This last home remedy may help because milk contains a bit of the amino acid tryptophan, which is known to produce drowsiness (turkey contains lots of tryptophan and that's supposed to explain why so many people nod off after a huge family Christmas or Thanksgiving meal). There may be something to this tryptophan business, because a recent study found that people given a milkshake with tryptophan before going to bed tended to feel more rested the next day, indicating they may have had a good night's sleep.

Some people also swear by the supplement melatonin, but the jury and I are still out on how effective it is. I've tried melatonin on several occasions, and I have never found it to work for me. Besides, one study found that in some birds, melatonin can lead to shrunken gonads, and I don't know about you, but for me, all the sleep in the world isn't worth tinier testicles.

Then there's this strategy. According to advice from Professor Jim Horne of Loughborough University of Technology in the UK, as reported in the London *Times,* warming the brain by increasing its visual workload in the daytime helps people sleep better. In other words, anything that makes the visual part of your brain work more, such as window shopping, Horne suggests, will help you sleep. Before you dismiss this suggestion as nonsense, let me tell you that I know at least one woman for whom this strategy works so well that she doesn't stop at the window, she actually goes into the store to shop to help herself sleep, and as far as I can judge, she always sleeps better than I do that night. Horne says that his theory that warming the brain helps you sleep better may also explain why sitting in a nice, hot bath is such an effective sleep remedy, especially, I suppose, in those people whose brain is situated where they sit.

Despite all those stratagies and remedies, surveys reveal that over one-third of North Americans still complain of chronic sleep problems. Why? Often, it's because they have another health condition that interferes with their ability to either fall asleep or stay asleep after nodding off.

There are now over eighty recognized sleep disorders, ranging from restless leg syndrome to chronic pain syndromes to menopause-related sleep disturbances to insomnia caused by an inability to fall asleep to insomnia from jolting awake prematurely several hours after going to bed. The point is that if you are developing a sleep problem, it's important to get it diagnosed properly and not just treat it as something that will pass. It may pass, as is the case usually with insomnia caused by a temporary worry about something, but it may also become chronic, and often the earlier you jump on these problems, the easier they are to treat.

What about sleeping pills? I have no hesitation in advising anyone with a case of acute insomnia to take a sleeping medication, even several times in a row during a particularly bad week, as when your kid suddenly returns home from school, at the age of thirty—to stay—with his family and three dogs. They are quick-acting and effective, and the shorter-acting ones do not lead to next-day drowsiness in most people. The problem with all these drugs, however, is that it is easy to become reliant on them. This is mostly a problem with the benzodiazepines (triazolam, temazepam, and several others) rather than with the newer non-addicting, central nervous system depressants (zolpidem and zopiclone), but it's my belief that even non-addicting drugs can become habit forming if you begin to believe you can't function without them. So never take sedatives or hypnotics for more than a few days in a row without having a chat with your physician about what else you can do to ease your problem, such as changing the locks on your front door. It is also important to be aware that some sleeping pills, especially the longer-acting ones, can produce sleepiness the next day and a consequent increased risk of accidents. Also, with some drugs, rebound insomnia can become a problem after prolonged use.

A quick few words about those special sleep-related problems, snoring and sleep apnea. Snoring occurs when air moves over an obstruction or through a narrowed channel. Thus, anything that lessens muscle tone in the neck and throat and allows the tissues to collapse more can make snoring worse, factors such as:

- being sedentary and weak-muscled
- being older
- being obese
- having allergies
- drinking alcohol

- using tranquillizers or drugs with a sedating effect, including some antihistamines
- having large tonsils and adenoids
- having a large uvula, nasal polyps, or a large tongue

Although traditionally considered to be a benign condition that is merely fodder for jokes, snoring is now known to be associated with several potential negative consequences (high blood pressure, diabetes, strokes, chronic headaches), not the least, of course, being the harm it brings to many relationships.

The treatment of snoring starts with removing the snorer to another bedroom. This usually solves the problem instantly for the bedmate. For the snorer, it's more advisable to begin by attacking any known contributing factor, such as minimizing the use of alcohol. Other strategies include elevating the head of the bed (the more upright you are, the less the tissues collapse, although many heavy snorers can sleep and snore just as well standing up), and using gadgets or reminders or strategies that lead to frequent changes of position, especially those that get the snorer off his back (my wife, for example, routinely kicks me during the night, and I really resent that, mostly because I don't snore). As well, mouth appliances that are worn at night and which realign the jaw to change the airflow through the throat seem to be successful in some people.

If all else fails, you might try one of those surgical techniques to remove the uvula and shrink the tissues at the back of the throat, but be aware that the long-term consequences of these procedures have still not been established. And finally, for women reading this, you can always try a husbandectomy.

In sleep apnea, which affects about 4 per cent of loud snorers, snoring is associated with a cessation in breathing for a period ranging from a few seconds to as long as ninety seconds on several and often many occasions a night. Several studies have linked sleep apnea to a higher risk of stroke and heart attack, especially in middle age, and happily, other studies are beginning to show that proper treatment of sleep apnea can mitigate those risks. Risk factors for sleep apnea include chronic loud snoring, obesity, and high blood pressure. You should suspect that you might have sleep apnea if 1) a bedmate tells you that when you sleep you sound like a sputtering eighteen-wheeler trying to rev its motor, and 2) you also suffer from such sleep-loss-related symptoms as:

- daytime fatigue
- excessive sleepiness
- memory impairment
- chronic morning headaches
- a recurrent tendency to crash your car

Sleep apnea is best diagnosed in a sleep lab and not by a wife.

Treatment starts with losing weight if you happen to be overweight, and minimizing the use of alcohol and sedatives. More active therapy consists of continuous positive airway pressure (CPAP) devices, which are worn at night and deliver a stream of air to the nose or mouth, and sometimes surgery.

As a final note, the benefits of getting sleep apnea properly diagnosed and treated are substantial. You not only reduce your risk of dying, you may also end up having more sex, at least according to one study that showed that men who had their sleep apnea taken care of ended up having way more sex as a result, probably because they had way more energy. I suppose, though, that they first had to take off those CPAP devices. Although maybe not.

Smoking

If you are a smoker and you decide to make only one change in your life to improve your chances of living long enough to witness Bob Geldof and Bono giving all their own money away (well, that might be asking a bit too much), give up smoking, man. According to a recent excellent review, quitting smoking can add up to ten years to a smoker's life, and the earlier you quit, the more time you add. In fact, if you quit early enough, your life expectancy becomes the same as that of a nonsmoker. Stopping smoking even at age sixty could still add nearly three years to life expectancy.

And the great thing is that the benefits kick in very quickly. As soon as one day after quitting, some experts say that your heart attack risk starts to fall, and after two weeks, the risk of clotting is significantly reduced. After one year, lung function has improved, lung-related symptoms such as coughing start to go away, and the risk of heart disease is cut in half, and within ten to fifteen years, most smoking-related risks (but not the excess risk of cancer) are back to normal.

And if you don't stop? A Canadian study found that smoking as few as three cigarettes a day wipes out the cardio-protective effects of ASA and two-thirds of the protective effect of taking cholesterol-lowering drugs. In other words, if you smoke, no matter what else you do, you are killing yourself much more rapidly than nature intended.

Smoking can kill you in several dozen ways, and you should know that it's working on each of those killer tracks simultaneously even as you sit there reading this. But if you give up smoking, it's not only yourself you will be helping by significantly reducing your risks of dying from all sorts of illnesses (heart attack and stroke, many forms of cancer, and such undignified diseases as terminal emphysema), you will also be helping all the newborns and infants and toddlers and even adults around you by minimizing their risk of secondhand smoke–related diseases.

Are there any secret miracle methods for quitting smoking? No. You have to want to quit, and if you want to badly enough, any of the plethora of stop-smoking aids out there—patches, gum, pills, counselling, cold turkey, acupuncture—will probably work equally well. Also, remember that you should never give up trying to quit. The average smoker makes eight attempts to quit before finally succeeding. And that's just an average, so you can bet that some people have made fifteen or maybe even twenty attempts before successfully giving up their dreadful habit. But succeed they did, and so can you.

I know how hard it is to give up smoking, I know how the tobacco companies have conspired to keep you addicted, I know how difficult your life is going to be for a few weeks or maybe even months, I know of the overheated claims that tobacco addiction is harder to beat than heroin addiction. But c'mon! Gimme a break! You're not a kid anymore, you have surely dealt with more difficult matters, and if you haven't then you certainly will pretty soon, and this task should be not much harder for the average man to deal with than most of the other difficult issues in life. Just give it up. It's time.

And best of all, when you finally quit, you will also be giving the finger to those damnable tobacco honchos who got you addicted in the first place. Wouldn't you just love to be part of a major movement that one day soon puts a couple of tobacco companies out of the death business?

{8}

PLAN C: PSYCHOLOGICAL HEALTH—GETTING YOUR HEAD AROUND IT

• • •

I know what men want. Men want to be really,
really close to someone who will leave them alone.

ELAYNE BOOSLER

When you are dissatisfied and would
like to go back to youth, think of Algebra.

WILL ROGERS

Better yet, don't.

ART HISTER

If you've read this far (and of course you have because here you are, mate), you will no doubt have noticed that I suffer from many of the health problems that I've mentioned up to this point, which, by the way, is also the reason that I was such a popular doctor. (Yes, I was popular, no matter what some of those close to me might want to tell you—she was never in my office so how would she know?) You see, for nearly every complaint that came my way in my practising days, I was nearly always able to cut the patient off within thirty seconds max (often within fifteen if they were slow talkers) by telling them, "Hey, you know? I've got exactly the same thing you've got. Only mine is way worse than yours. Next." My patients loved those laments of mine for some reason, and they kept coming back to visit me in droves, probably in part to see if they could one-up me the next time they came in. Rarely did, though.

So, dear reader, after advising you to skip the next bit if you have a delicate "moogen" (Yiddish for digestive system, but as with all Yiddishisms, it means so much more than just a stomach and bowels), which might be upset by more yucky stuff than you want to know about me, I must admit that I have:

- high cholesterol
- pretty severe gastroesophageal reflux disease
- a woeful back (although it's acting up much less often than it used to thanks to the abs I've developed from all those crunches I'm now doing regularly, although on the downside, those crunches, like the Pilates I used to do, have markedly worsened my reflux; you think I should try kabala next?)
- disc deterioration in my neck with an intermittently numb right forearm
- the remnants of bilateral partially frozen shoulders
- a chronically aching right hamstring
- the world's worst gums (which has also led me to discover the world's second unfunniest dentist, behind only Eugene Levy in *Waiting for Guffman*)
- had my knees scoped twice to get rid of torn cartilage
- had several bowel polyps removed (I warned you this wasn't going to be pleasant, didn't I?) and have to get scoped (that's that colonoscopy thing) regularly
- suffered one episode of acute, severe, viselike chest pain (although luckily, it does not seem to have been heart-related; I'm still here, eh?)

Some will also want to tell you that I have the clear beginnings of brain deterioration, but I dispute that mainly because I've always been like this.

In addition, there is the stuff I didn't cover in this book, such as my awful allergies, my asthma, my celiac disease, my psoriasis, my rectal bleeding, and my arteriovenous malformation, which is all I'm going to reveal here because some of this stuff is really better kept private. ("Yah, like what?" my wife challenged when she read this. You don't want to know, believe me.)

So, how, you wonder, do I deal with all that physical misfortune? With lots and lots of pills, of course. Hey, just kidding! Those medications only augment my constantly sunny disposition, and no more. Actually, I dislike taking medication so I take very few drugs apart from those that keep a dyspeptic lid on my GERD and control my asthma and my abnormal cholesterol levels. Instead, I prefer to deal with my rather imperfect body mostly by not worrying about any of my problems too much, which is often much more easily said than done, especially when I can't sleep at night because that GERD is giving me heartburn and that arteriovenous malformation is booming out a Scottish tattoo in my ear. Happily, though, I've also been blessed with a pretty upbeat outlook on life, or as my wife likes to tell people who ask why I'm always smiling so much, "Too dumb to know he should be unhappy."

Many midlife men, however, are not as fortunate, and they suffer from any one of a number of psychological problems, although two stand out for me: depression and excess stress.

So, for once, this chapter is going to be about medical conditions I don't suffer from, but which are common in midlifers nonetheless.

Depression

Although the numbers vary significantly in studies because of how depression is defined and diagnosed, it is generally agreed that about 15 per cent of North American adults suffer from depression at some point in their lives, a steep rise over the last half-century. And North Americans are certainly not unique in their susceptibility to mood disorders because depression seems to be sharply increasing all around the world. In fact, WHO has estimated that by the year 2020, depression will be the second leading cause of chronic disability and time lost from work. The leading cause? Laziness, of course. Just kidding. It's actually cardiovascular disease—except in France, bien sur, where it really is laziness. I mean, ever try to get a French plumber to fix the overflow in your hotel room? "Non, non, non. Pas possible. Peut-être, Doctor Hister, July 2007. Je regrette, mais c'est pas grand chose, eh, because you can utiliser ze toilette in ze café. Next block."

So who gets depressed? That's easy: anyone can get depressed, although certain factors are clearly linked to a higher risk:

- having been previously diagnosed with depression
- having a family history of depression
- suffering from some metabolic illnesses such as thyroid disease and diabetes
- taking any one of several medications, including calcium channel blockers, statins, amphetamines, anabolic steroids, and others
- suffering from a sleep disturbance, which, interestingly, can be either the symptom of a mood disorder (depression is notorious for interfering with proper sleep—see below) or the cause of one: thus, an American study found that male medical students who had trouble sleeping were twice as likely to be diagnosed with depression thirty years later than their peers who, like me as an intern, had absolutely no trouble falling asleep while reading X-rays and ECGs or listening to a hypochondriac's list of complaints at three A.M.

One of the facts about depression that may surprise you is that depression is not just a psychological or mental health problem but that it can have major physical consequences, too. Thus, studies have linked depression to many conditions, including higher rates of heart attack, stroke, irregular heart rhythm, high blood pressure, diabetes, and dementia.

Quite a list, and one that should help make clear why depression is related to a significantly higher risk of death. Unfortunately, what is not nearly as clear is whether treating depression adequately will lower most of those risks substantially. Take the excess risk of heart disease linked to depression, for example. Although it is probable that once someone is successfully treated for depression, he is more likely, at the very least, to try to follow some of the lifestyle habits (not smoking, eating better, doing some exercise) that would lower his subsequent risk of heart disease than if he stayed depressed, it has been quite difficult to substantiate in rigorous studies that such changes actually improve cardiac outcomes.

So what happens in depression? Again, despite all the research, no one knows for sure, mainly because it's hard to get a good peek into the brain (at least while a person is alive). That said, we do know that depression involves very important changes in brain chemistry, most notably changes in the levels and actions of neurotransmitters such as serotonin and norepinephrine. That is clearly not the complete answer, however, or else the SSRI (selective serotonin reuptake inhibitor) antidepressants such as fluoxetine (Prozac) and paroxetine (Paxil) would cure nearly everyone, yet they obviously don't. In fact, there is a growing debate about whether such antidepressants even work at all (see below).

Symptoms

Although depression can produce any symptoms whatsoever (often by aggravating underlying concomitant health problems), a major review of depression summarized the more common symptoms as:

- a depressed or irritable mood most of the day, nearly every day
- a diminished interest or pleasure in most activities
- significant weight loss or weight gain
- insomnia or sleeping too much nearly every day
- agitation or sluggishness most of the time
- fatigue or loss of energy most of the time
- intense feelings of worthlessness

- a drop in ability to concentrate
- indecisiveness
- recurrent thoughts of death or suicide

But that's certainly not all. To this list you can also add fairly common features of depression such as loss of appetite and sex drive, and an inability to experience pleasure, although I must point out that an inability to experience, or at least express, pleasure and happiness is clearly not a sine qua non of depression since that symptom (i.e., anti-hedonism) is palpably present in nearly every thirty-something, and it's doubtful, I think, that an entire generation could be depressed. In other words, anti-hedonism is often just an attitude thing. Right, dude? Whatever.

Some depressives also exhibit a heightened level of anxiety, with symptoms such as palpitations, sweating, agitation, phobias, fears, and worries—in short, all the signs a Jewish mother exhibits when her thirty-year-old son is two minutes late coming home. On Saturday afternoon. From synagogue. One block away. With his wife.

It's also important to point out that you don't have to have all of these features to be diagnosed with depression, although the more of them you have, the more likely that diagnosis becomes.

Although that list of symptoms is quite substantial and makes it seem as if a diagnosis of depression should be a slam-dunk, the signs and symptoms of depression are often quite subtle, and consequently, depression often goes unnoticed or unacknowledged for a long time, even years. One survey found, for example, that only one in four depressed people has received therapy, in large part because so many patients don't admit their symptoms or fears to their doctors. Why are people much less likely to admit to feelings of depression than they are to admit to suffering from physical ailments? Lots of reasons.

For a start, even though depression, like erectile dysfunction, has come some way out of its long-tenanted closet, there is still a huge stigma associated with a diagnosis of depression, as well as potential penalties. Thus, many depressed people probably don't come forward for treatment because they worry about the effects a diagnosis of depression might have either on their job (prospects for promotion, for example) or on their rights to both health and life insurance. Also, some depressed people (read: men) often don't think their symptoms need treatment. Or they believe that these lousy feelings will dissipate over time no matter what they do. Or they feel ashamed of their problem and feel they should be able to deal with their "head space" with simple willpower. Moreover, many depressives still feel that health professionals can offer them little in the way of therapy aside from a lifetime's worth of drugs, which they are reluctant to take.

Even when depression is easily recognized and acknowledged, however, it is often treated inadequately. According to an expert American panel, fewer than one-third of depressed patients who are given antidepressants take a high enough dose to get the full benefits of their medication. As well, studies indicate that 40 per cent of people who committed suicide had visited their family doctor in the month before they took their own lives. Why do we do such a poor job of treating depression adequately? Besides the questions that surround the effectiveness of treatments for depression (see below), one important reason for this failure is that patients and doctors often just don't communicate well about this illness. In fact, in a recent survey, more than 75 per cent of depressed patients felt their depression was poorly controlled, and more than 50 per cent had stopped their medications because of side effects, yet many of these people had not discussed their problems with their doctors.

So if you take nothing else from this discussion, take at least this: if you are depressed, it's unlikely that you will get better on your own, no matter what some Hollywood celebrity masquerading as a mental health expert might tell you, and the road to better health must start with your admission—to yourself, to your significant other or family members or friends, and to your doctor—of your condition.

The curious thing about depression, though, is that it isn't only underdiagnosed and undertreated. Paradoxically, there has also been a strong tendency to overdiagnose depression and to overuse therapies, most significantly medications. This will be anathema to that army of interventionists out there who believe that every tic needs a tweaking and that every droop needs a drug, but hey, folks, it's actually normal not to feel happy all the time, and feeling low occasionally is not a mental health problem that requires intervention. In fact, I would argue that it's actually good for you to experience low moods from time to time simply because it helps you appreciate life's highs more. Yet, ever since Prozac hit the markets, we have witnessed a vocal movement, most prominently in the intervention-happy U.S., that claims that nearly all of us require some form of treatment, if not permanently, then at least occasionally. Thus, a recent expert panel of American physicians concluded that the majority of the population suffers from some form of mental illness (except, I suppose, the members of the panel), which, if you ask me, is absolutely nutso (to use a technical term), even in America. Just because Paxil and Prozac can help some people with depression (and there is much debate even about that simple claim) does not mean that everyone should automatically start taking one of them when they're feeling a bit down, and you should never allow yourself to be pushed into taking an antidepressant just because you're not feeling up to par and someone thinks it might help.

Treatment

The best treatment for depression is clearly to prevent it in the first place. And happily, that can be done to a certain extent, perhaps through diet, and more probably with exercise. Thus, a higher intake of fish has been linked to a lower incidence of depression, and should always be encouraged in people at high risk. Fish oils probably exert their effect because of their potent anti-inflammatory properties, since inflammation is now thought to play a role in this condition (as it seems to in so many others). A diet high in fruits and veggies has also been linked to a lower risk of depression, although before you rush out to corner your corner store's supply of canned herring and eggplant, be aware that this mitigating effect of diet on depression may only be a reflection of the fact that people who eat better are less at risk for depression to begin with.

So what about exercise? Although one large American study on doctors failed to find that exercise prevented depression, exercise has been linked in many other studies to both a lowered risk of becoming depressed in the first place and to improvement in symptoms of depression that do come on. Thus, one lovely sixteen-week study found that even in people diagnosed with moderate-to-severe depression, a good exercise regimen (thirty to fifty minutes five times a week) worked as well as the best medications. Besides, exercise has never been linked to making depression worse, so if you're trying to stave off depression, or even if you're already depressed, always consider doing some exercise as a first step in self-treatment. And honestly, wouldn't you rather pump iron than pop Prozac?

If exercise is not your bag, however, you and your doctor will then need to turn to some other form of therapy based on his and especially your prejudices. And make no mistake, prejudice—or "patient choice" as it's more commonly called these days when patients are "clients" and doctors are "health providers"—is a key factor in determining the effectiveness of a particular treatment for depression. In fact, a recent study concluded that patient choice, a factor that is often very much influenced by the treating physician, is probably the most important factor in how well a therapy will work for that patient.

Although there are as many depression therapies as there are people who promise you that they can make you feel better if only you follow what they prescribe, the most commonly used therapies can be broken into two broad categories: talking and taking, whose practitioners, naturally enough, can be called talkers or takers.

Talkers believe that most cases of depression should be treated with psychotherapy. In support of this view, a recent good study has concluded that a short course of cognitive behaviour therapy from a trained therapist works as well as medication in alleviating most cases of depression.

A taker, by contrast, will pooh-pooh such claims and will choose instead to dispense his cure from the insides of a capsule rather than via the insights of a bearded therapist. I call them takers, by the way, in honour of my mom, who, whenever she's cooked something for me that is "guaranteed, Arthur, to make you feel better" (never does, though), sings me a constant refrain of "Take, take, take." (It's a cover version of an old James Brown number.)

Does it really matter which of these broad approaches you try first? Yes and no. Yes, because as stated earlier, your prejudice is key in helping you get better. So if, on the one hand, you're like most of my old patients and very reluctant to take drugs (prescribed ones, at any rate), then you're clearly more likely to get better quickly if you start with counselling instead of capsules. If, on the other hand, the thought of going to a therapist who will question you about matters you'd rather not fess up about fills you with dread (or worse, makes you burst out laughing), then I'd suggest you start with some pills and see where that gets you.

And for many reasons (cost, ease of access, convenience, privacy, etc.), taking some type of medication is by far the preferred current first-attempt route, and one of the most popular drugs to start with is St. John's wort. In several widely reported studies, mostly from Europe, where this herb has been used for over two hundred years, St. John's wort has been found to be as effective as synthetic antidepressants for all degrees of depression, that is, mild, moderate, and even severe (although, to be fair, other studies have disputed these claims). Be aware, though, that despite being a herb, St. John's wort is a drug (hey, that's why it may work) and thus has important potential side effects and can produce interactions with other drugs, even with birth control pills. Also, as I write this, there is still no standardization applied to herbal products, so you can never really know when you buy St. John's wort that you're actually getting what you paid for. Not only can manufacturers cheat on what they put into those bottles, even when it's definitely St. John's wort in the bottle, they could still have cheated or erred (same thing, often) on the strength of the formulation. Even though it's available over-the-counter, I would still suggest that you never take St. John's wort without at the very least telling your doctor about it. And make sure to monitor your progress honestly.

When it comes to manufactured medications, there is a slew of synthetic antidepressants to choose from, although the newer SSRIs and SNRIs (serotonin and norepinephrine reuptake inhibitors) have largely replaced the older tricyclics as drugs of first choice. These drugs boost the levels of neurotransmitters in the brain by allowing them to circulate longer. These drugs seem to be somewhat effective (though not nearly as effective, I think, as most proponents claim; they probably work in some subpopulations better than in others, but alas! we still don't know who will respond best to them), they are relatively well tolerated (see potential side effects below), and for some people such as heart patients, they appear to be safer than the tricyclics. That's the (limited) positives, although for the right person, those probably outweigh the potential list of negatives, which is a substantial one.

For a start, these drugs can produce lots of side effects, and among the more common and significant ones, are the twin devils of sleep disturbance and sexual dysfunction, the latter often in the forms of decreased libido and "delayed orgasm." For example, a Dutch study found that antidepressant drugs can "seriously" delay male orgasm. Specifically, time to orgasm (that's two nouns, by the way, not a noun and a verb) was delayed up to eight times longer, long enough, say the researchers, to "disrupt" intercourse, although I figure that most women would be only too happy to have intercourse "disrupted" to eight times its normal length, because that way total time from "What about it?" to "Good night, then" might actually approach several minutes.

Also, when you discontinue your SSRI medication, you may suffer withdrawal effects such as nausea, dizziness, tremor, anxiety, and palpitations, and although these symptoms can often be minimized by gradually tapering the dose, some people develop severe symptoms and find it very difficult to come off some of these drugs. As well, SSRI antidepressants have been linked to higher risks of bleeding from the gastrointestinal tract, especially in the elderly, so the combination of a nonsteroidal anti-inflammatory drug and an SSRI drug is something you'd really like to avoid, especially in the long term. And finally, and perhaps most troubling, these drugs have been linked to higher rates of suicide. This seems to be especially a problem in kids in whom such antidepressants must be used with great caution. But although this link has been most prominently played up in kids, some experts believe the same effect can—and does—happen on occasion in adults, too.

You should also know that antidepressants don't kick in for at least several days and may take up to several weeks to prove effective. And once you decide to take them, you should continue taking them long enough to let them do all they are meant to do, usually a period of several months. Furthermore, if you have been diagnosed with recurring depression, many experts believe that you should stay on antidepressants for life, although I can't really see why you shouldn't try to take a holiday from drugs whenever you think the time is propitious, albeit after consultation with your doctor. Or better yet, why not get him to prescribe you a placebo instead (although he clearly can't tell you that's what you're getting) since many studies have found that placebos are nearly as effective as SSRI antidepressants.

So here's that old bottom line again: there is no formula to help you decide what to do, although if you're depressed, the most important thing is to get better. So if you believe in medication, and if you're honest about how you're doing, it's probably worth risking the potential downsides of these drugs, for a while at least. Your call, though.

Among the myriad other therapies that have been touted for depression are sleep-deprivation therapy, that is, not being allowed to sleep, thus presumably resetting the biological clock and the brain's neurotransmitters (although if sleep deprivation is so good at preventing depression, why is postpartum depression often so difficult to deal with?); dance therapy (the effectiveness of this approach probably depends on who your dance partner happens to be); narrative therapy, or telling your story to others (not for everyone, though; in a men's group I once belonged to—don't ask, I was younger—one guy admitted that his biggest fear was boring people, a fear that was confirmed by the two guys who had clearly fallen asleep while he was talking); acupuncture; art therapy; writing therapy; music therapy (although I'd suggest that you don't start with rap songs); rolfing; implanted devices that stimulate the vagus nerve (some even stimulate areas of the brain); and this book.

Stress

Excess stress is rampant. According to one survey, two thirds of Americans feel stressed out at least once a week, and that's just the over-the-top I-can't-manage-anymore-cuz-it's-all-just-wearing-me-down-so-much-that-I-better-eat-another-tub-of-Ben-and-Jerry's-Cherry-Garcia kind of stress, which has, of course, been linked to numerous potential health problems (see below). The more niggling, one-off, gee-I-hope-the-test-comes-back-normal-because-I-don't-know-what-I'm-gonna-tell-what's-her-name kind of stress is much more prevalent, and it can affect you adversely as well.

Consequences

So what can chronic stress do to you? Far too much, I'm afraid. Some of the common and serious health problems that are related to excess stress include:

- premature aging
- heart attacks
- strokes
- heart rhythm abnormalities
- cardiac ischemia, or decreased blood flow to heart tissue
- cardiac-associated sudden death
- high blood pressure
- diabetes
- erectile dysfunction (Hey, the surprise would be if ED and stress weren't connected.)
- depression and suicide
- gastroesophageal reflux

Stress may even be associated with a higher rate of some cancers, although, to be fair, there is still a fierce debate going on among the experts about whether stress can directly cause malignancy. All the experts do agree on one thing, however, and that is that no one who comes down with cancer should ever feel that they brought the malignancy on themselves by becoming too stressed, although unhappily, many cancer patients still do blame themselves for their cancer.

Chronic stress also:

- causes blood platelets to become stickier, thus leading to more clots
- produces deleterious changes in inflammatory proteins

- slows the healing of wounds
- impairs immunity
- impairs the blood-brain barrier (this might—might—even be related to a higher risk of problems such as dementia)
- increases that dreaded abdominal fat storage
- interrupts testosterone production (perhaps that's why some men's voices go up so high when they're stressed; when, for example, I answer the phone and I realize that it's one of those telephone solicitation people, nearly all of them immediately ask if they can talk to my daddy instead of me; I invariably hand the phone to my wife, and no one has ever called back)
- lowers sperm counts
- impairs memory and problem-solving abilities
- reduces the ability to learn new tasks
- leaves you more open to coming down with infections (although this one is also the subject of much debate since some studies show that flu shots don't work as well if you get them when you're stressed while others have found that getting a flu shot while under a bit of stress enhances the immune response to the shot)

Moreover, stress probably also affects us, perhaps especially men, in subtle ways that we are not yet completely aware of. It certainly has some subtle effects in animals. For example, when a male cichlid fish is under chronic high stress, he fails to develop the "bright, war-like colors, the extra muscles and the [ohmygawd!] fully mature sex organs" he is naturally prone to develop. So what are your war-like colours like, bro? Faded to white? Notice, also, that I didn't ask about your fully mature gonads because it's really none of my business.

What We Know about Stress

What's so curious about these negative consequences of stress is that a stress reaction started out as something very useful, and in its place it still is. That old fight-or-flight reaction in response to some perceived danger or threat to your well-being—a marauding sabre-toothed tiger, for example, or an apple-bearing snake—has served from the beginning of our bipedal existence as a very useful, often lifesaving response. Back on the savanna, when a tiger came around to mull over which one of our ancestors he would prefer for lunch, it was useful, if not essential, for each of those endangered beings to instantly secrete a flood of hormones, which in turn mobilized and jump-started his brain and other neurological and endocrine systems to get him the hell out of there, a very good thing for him and an even better one for us or else none of us would be here. Thus, those people who mounted a strong stress response when tigers prowled lived to pass on their DNA, while those who manifested little anxiety or worry at the sight of "Oh, what a cute large kitty, and so many stripes, too!" have no descendants, and their genes are no longer with us.

Today we may not have to flee from tigers, but our ancestors' legacy remains. Our modern-day hero, faced with a tiger equivalent—another driver cutting him off, for example, or a spouse who insists on painting the house again even though it was re-painted only twelve years ago—is still able to mount an instant put-em-up-or-I'm-outta-here stress response and jump-start his biochemical and neurological systems.

Happily, each individual stress reaction is unlikely to do us much harm, although as we all know from ready examples among our acquaintances an acutely stressful event can result in adverse consequences to the heart and sometimes even sudden cardiac death. ("Poor Melvin. Did you hear, Bob? Came home suddenly, found his wife in bed with his partner, and pffft. Gone. Left her a fortune. What a pity." "Yes, Charles. What did you say her number is?") For example, managers who fire someone double their risk of suffering a heart attack for the week after they sack the employee (curiously, there was no word in this study on what the employees may have suffered). Also, the rate of cardiac events, heart rhythm abnormalities, and even sudden death has been shown to rise significantly among members of communities subject to terrorist attacks, such as the residents of New York City post 9/11. But it's not just root-causes-justify-murder terrorists who raise one's risk of heart attack. So can down-home, old-line terrorists such as, for example, your algebra teacher (square-root causes?). Thus, one study found that simply asking high-risk men to do a difficult math problem was enough to trigger a potentially life-threatening abnormal heart rhythm in some of them.

But given how many acutely stressful events we are prone to on a regular basis, it's clear that most of the time we handle sudden acute stress without any deleterious consequences. It's chronic stress that's the real problem for most of us because repeated pulses of stress hormones wear down our bodies and can lead to all those negative effects that were mentioned earlier.

Clearly, though, chronic stress can and does affect each of us to a different extent, especially in its effects on the cardiovascular system. Take, for example, a study that found that stressed-out Finnish men who don't ski-jump have much higher rates of coronary heart disease than those who do. Why? Mainly, of course, because of the constant ribbing and ostracism the non-jumpers face from the rest of the nation. Just kidding, of course, because there really are no Finns who don't ski-jump. What this study actually concluded is that some Finnish men were much more likely to react to stress by developing coronary heart disease than were other Finnish men. Same type of guy, same level of stress, different effects on the heart.

So the really big question is: why do some men's cardiovascular systems react to stress in a worse fashion than do others? Genetics and early environment are certainly vital factors, although, sadly, we still don't know nearly as much about their influence as we should. But what we do know is not that comforting. For example, several studies done on rodents have shown that rats and mice respond to stressful events in their adult lives based in large part on how well nurtured they have been by their mothers as infants. The same is very likely true in humans, too. It certainly would explain a lot about me, for example. You see, my dad apparently never put me down when I was a baby (a period that lasted till I was eighteen years old), which has probably contributed greatly to making me feel very secure as an adult, although the downside is that I'm scared to death that men with two-day-old growths on their faces will pick me up and hold me tight.

Another key factor in our ability to deal with stress is our social and economic environment. After all, it's just common sense that the less you have to worry about from a financial and social and employment perspective, the happier and less worried you will be (unless, of course, you're a Jewish mother, when the happier you are, the more you will worry about why you're so happy). Thus, a Centers for Disease Control report from the U.S. determined that the lowest rates of mental stress were found in employed, educated, middle-class, middle-aged Americans, although curiously the overall lowest rates were reported by sixty-five-year-old men living in South Dakota. (That's still not enough reason to move to Pierre, though.)

Another key factor in determining how we deal with stress is psychological make-up or personality type, and this has many dimensions. For a start there's that grand fissure between Type A and Type B personalities. Thus, as most of you are no doubt aware, Type A people are awful, aggressive, opinionated, impatient individuals (generally of the male persuasion) with a consequent terrible prognosis (ha, ha, on them), while Type B folks are gentle, kind, and patient hummingbirds who are likely to live forever as a result of their placidity. This is all based on much-hyped work done several decades ago by some American researchers, who identified having a Type A personality as an important link to a significantly higher risk of heart attacks from stress. According to that early research, a Type A man—a driven and intense individual who rudely cuts into line, finishes other people's sentences for them, and volubly counts the number of items other shoppers have in their baskets in the express check-out line (you have no idea, by the way, how many people with too many items try to sneak into those express lines)—is much more at risk, these researchers claimed, of heart attack compared with his more laid-back "Hey, no worries, man, take your 60 items through ahead of me in the express line and anyone else wanna push in front, too?" Type B brother. This Type A–Type B dichotomy was the accepted template for many years, which was, of course, very bad news and indicated a very dire prognosis for quintessential Type As, such as your "Hey-buddy-that's-ten-items-you-have-there-and-this-line-is-for-nine-items-max-can't-you-read-the-signs" author.

But these are much happier days for this prototypical don't-interrupt-me-while-I'm-interrupting-you guy because it has now become clear that although some Type A men are indeed at much higher risk of calamitous cardiac consequences, many, probably most, Type A men live just as long and as well as their Type B bros. So, over the last few years, the experts have begun to focus on certain attitudes or features of personality as being much more predictive of an increased risk of heart attack than the overall simple categorization into Type A and Type B.

To that end, they have singled out hostility as a particularly important personality trait linked to a higher risk of a heart attack from stress. In fact, one provocative study concluded that hostility is a better measure of eventual heart health than any other gauge, including cholesterol levels and blood pressure. So how the hell do they describe a hostile man, many of you are probably growling at your spouse who is reading this part to you because you're too upset to read it yourself? They describe him as a distrustful man who is not only quick to become angry but who is also more likely to act on his anger—a lane-changing horn honker, in other words. Anyone you know, by the way? Hey, take it easy. I was just asking, that's all.

Sadly, I think these mavens may be on to something for once. So, leaving aside the issue that really burns me up—namely, how so-called experts have the chutzpah to label a great driver like me a "hostile person"—I must admit, although it makes my blood boil to do so, that there is some good evidence that being hostile is bad for you, especially when you're a younger dude. Thus, compared with their more accommodating, even-tempered, and impossibly naïve brothers, hostile males have been found to:

- have lower HDL and higher LDL cholesterol levels at age nineteen
- suffer from more "bad habits," such as smoking and excess alcohol intake, at age forty-two
- have higher blood pressures in midlife even during sleep
- be prone to an increased risk of death from all causes

In fact, one study even concluded that the reason we can only link these poor health consequences to hostility in young adulthood and middle age and not in older guys is simply because there are so few older hostile men left alive to study. Oh, yeah? So how come the world is so full of crusty old farts, eh?

Along similar lines of trying to find specific personality traits to focus on when assessing cardiovascular risks, some researchers have proposed a subcategory under "hostility"—what they call "dominance"—as a particularly toxic character trait. Thus, a study from Duke University found that dominant men—guys who always feel compelled to be the centre of what's going on (moi?) and who repeatedly interrupt conversations—were 60 per cent more likely to die during the twenty-two-year study than were their less intrusive brothers.

Another personality trait that has been linked to poorer outcomes is called time/urgency impatience (TUI), or what I call "the waiting husband syndrome" in which no one, but especially one's wife, is ever ready on time for anything, anywhere. Studies have found that even young people with TUI are much more likely to have high blood pressure than their ever-late brothers. TUI is probably also partially behind the consistent finding that commuting through heavy traffic is linked to a much higher risk of heart attack (and incidentally why so many husbands die so much sooner than their wives—see Chapter 6).

Another aspect of psychological make-up linked to poorer health is plain old excess worrying, not the "Oh, gee, I can't decide whether to have a latte or a cappuccino" kind of concern (and how come, I want to know, that's always a major dilemma for the woman holding up the line in front of me at Starbucks—the same woman who then spends another two minutes deciding between a croissant and a scone, and who finally takes an extra five minutes to find the exact change in her wallet?), but rather the really serious kind of persistent excess worrying, what doctors refer to as chronic anxiety, but which Mel Brooks more accurately referred to as "High Anxiety." Thus, men who complain of being very anxious were found to be four to six times more likely to die from a sudden heart attack than their more laid-back brothers.

A particularly troubling type of anxiety seems to be manifested by men who suffer from what researchers called "heightened vigilance," or just being constantly tense about the potential dangers in one's environment—always watching out for ladders not to walk under, worrying about the effects shampoo can have on their sperm count, or in my case, being constantly on guard for one of my mother's famous double-ended questions. (An old joke: a Jewish son comes down to dinner wearing one of the two ties his mother gave him, and she asks, "So, Arthur, what's wrong with the other one? Arthur, stop yelling at me. You're too nervous.") Heightened vigilance has been linked to "heightened cardiovascular reactivity," which in turn raises the risk of heart attack and sudden death.

Bottom line: like your upbringing, your employment status, your level of education, and your genes, your personality, too, has a lot to do with how you handle stress and the effects that stress will exert on your health.

Reducing the Effects of Stress

Given that stress is so multi-factorial, the question many of you need to ask yourselves is, can I do anything to handle stress better? This is especially important given the fact that that by middle age all of you have developed certain techniques to help you deal with your stress load, techniques that you've either stumbled upon or have consciously developed because you felt they were best suited to you. And boy, do we ever have lots of techniques! Thus, some men pray, some men pay, some men play, some men golf (the preceding four go hand-in-hand in most duffers, by the way), some yell, some smoke, some drink, some run, some sit, some surf, some read, some meditate, some do yoga, some attend yoga classes just to watch (that can be dangerous), and on and on.

If these tactics work for you, by all means continue to use them (all except smoking and excess drinking, of course, and golf). If, however, you are not doing well, if you are feeling too stressed, if you are beginning to lose it or to burn out, if you or those who care for you perceive that you are not handling matters with your usual aplomb, then it's time to do something before the stress gets you.

There are literally thousands of stress-fighting strategies, techniques, and plans out there, and all of them probably work for some people, but I have only limited space, so here are a few worth mentioning:

- Start to do regular exercise, which in many studies has been shown to significantly reduce stress levels, assuming, that is, the concern about needing to do the exercise doesn't coincidentally raise your stress level instead. But if doing exercise does happen to make you more tense (when? what? for how long? etc.), just remember this: you don't really have to count every calorie and chart every second's effort and every biceps curl repetition to get the stress-busting benefits of working out. You're doing this to relax, guy, not to obsess. And if you happen to miss a workout or two, so be it, although make sure that you don't miss too many workouts with some simple precooked excuses (no time, too hot, too cold, too late, too early, too wet, etc.). I am as busy as anyone, yet I rarely excuse myself from my exercise classes because I know how much I need them to reduce my stress levels (and besides, I also pre-pay for those classes and you can only cancel them with twenty-four hours' notice, and there's no way I'm not going to get my full money's worth from those dudes).
- Sit down, preferably with your partner—that's the one who shares your bed, not your office (although if it's both, I think I know why you're so stressed)—and reassess your priorities. Everyone, even the president of the U.S., can make changes in his life to make it more stress-free if the stakes (divorce, for example, or nuclear conflagration) are high enough. Thus, to the extent you can, try to work fewer hours, or try to delegate unnecessary jobs, or try to say "no" more often to excessive demands, and so on. In other words, weigh your life as objectively as you can, and try to eliminate sources of extra pressure. This is far easier said than done, of course, although most midlifers I know and probably most midlifers who buy this book can in fact develop some strategies if they just want to enough. Delegating tasks, for example, is rather easy to do. (I mean, just ask my wife. Hey, only kidding. She doesn't actually delegate; she just pronounces.) Anyway, it's much easier to delegate once you accept that even though no one will ever do any job as well as you, you don't really have to do everything yourself and you can live with the results of an imperfect job.
- You might also try to get some friends, hard as that may be for some guys to do, because men who have no social and emotional support are more than twice as likely to die after a heart attack than those with a caring family and friends (see Chapter 10). You have to pick the right family and friends,

though, because conflict with close family members has been shown to set off stress reactions in heart disease patients. ("You want to me to sell the house and move to a home? Oy! All of sudden, I have chest pains.")

- You might also think of getting a pet, although for pretty obvious reasons, I strongly recommend starting with a bird or a worm, not a Doberman or pit bull. Studies show that caring for pets is very effective at helping lower stress levels. In fact, a provocative study from the University of Buffalo Medical School found that in times of high stress, even a supportive partner can't get your blood pressure and heart rate down as much as a pet can. On the negative side, a pet is much more likely to chew the furniture than a spouse or friends are.
- You might also consider buying any one of a host of books or visual aids that can teach you how to relax, such as a yoga DVD or *The Relaxation Response* by Herbert Benson, MD, or my other book, which, trust me, is even better than this one. And then there are all those pop psychology books that generally contain at least one or two ideas and strategies to consider, so pick up one of those best sellers and see what it can do for you. Besides, you'll get a good laugh out of most of them because those books are so funny in their earnestness and "capsulization" and attempts at universal meaning. (Hey, someone just moved my cheese while I was writing that.)

If you're one of those men who erupts easily, you should also work on your anger control, and please don't blow up at me for mentioning this, because I'm just trying to help. Why control your anger? Because the more stress you're under, the more angry outbursts you erupt with, and anger can kill you (not to mention that it can kill others, too). Thus, one study found that compared with their more placid brothers, the "angriest" men were significantly more likely to develop a dangerous abnormal heart rhythm and were also more likely to die during this ten-year-long study. Furthermore, sudden bursts of anger have been found to raise the risk of heart attack for up to two hours afterwards.

Now, most angry men don't really need expensive anger management classes, they just need to work more on their common anger-provoking triggers and responses to those triggers. So rather than blowing up the next time she insists there is an urgent need to add more shelves in the bedroom (and hey, what's wrong with boxes for underwear, anyway?), let her win the argument instead. And smile over your canned tuna as your dog contentedly digests the dinner steak he grabbed from your kitchen counter during the shelves discussion. Relax, mate. It's just not worth getting upset about such trivial matters.

Actually, since studies have shown that positive emotions are associated with a lower risk of heart problems, I suggest that you try to work on becoming even more broadminded and going the extra step, such as, for example, giving the dog another steak. And rather than just walking out of the room muttering to yourself about unneeded storage, why not instead ask your wife if she would like to go to a movie with (her words) the biggest moron in town? You'll not only be more likely to live longer, she might even forget about the shelves if you go to enough movies.

Finally, if despite your best efforts (you work out like a dog, dog it at work, own a dog, and do a daily "down dogs" when you feel angry), stress is still getting the better of you, you have to learn to reach out for help, a very unmacho thing to do, and something far too many men avoid until they've exploded. Now by "reaching out" I certainly don't mean that you have to put your arm around your best buddy's shoulder tonight, stare into his eyes, and murmur, "There's something I've been meaning to tell you, Jake," mainly because Jake will panic, spill his beer, and fly right out of there.

What I do mean is that if you are clearly paying a price for being under too much stress, you simply have to get up the guts to talk to someone about it, preferably a professional (bartenders and hookers are not the kind of professionals I mean). If you don't get some help, you run the great risk of getting those stress-related conditions mentioned earlier or of harming yourself by burning out (or if you're an American postal worker, harming others when you burn out), or worse, of starting to rely on inappropriate stress-relief strategies such as drinking too much or golfing excessively, terrible remedies for stress in that they invariably increase marital strife.

Unfortunately, many men have to overcome innate fears and prejudices before they can seek professional help, even for minor problems. Thus, one British study found that 42 per cent of British men, those guys famous for their stiff upper lips, would ignore symptoms until they were so acute that they could no longer manage on their own. In fact, over half of all the men surveyed viewed any sickness at all as a weakness, and you can well imagine that if they believe physical illness is a weakness, how much more likely they are to consider that to be true of psychological illness.

But that attitude also helps explain why men don't live as long as women. So guys: getting sick doesn't mean you're a weakling. Don't get me wrong, pal. I'm not saying you're not weak. I don't know you well enough to judge. I am saying, though, that when you get sick or when you feel overwhelmed, there's absolutely no shame and lots to gain from seeking professional help. Your kids' kids will thank me for this advice.

What will a professional do for you? If they're at all on the ball, at the very least they will direct you to a stress management program that's right for you. And stress management programs do work. One study showed, for example, that heart disease patients who learned to manage stress through biofeedback and relaxation were over 70 per cent less likely to have a heart attack than patients who received only standard medical care.

A health professional might also advise you to try some medication, often one of the SSRI antidepressants such as Paxil, which, according to one good review, appear to "reduce hostility and may even boost cooperative behavior," although I suppose that you have to cooperate enough to take the bloody pill in the first place. Oops! Must be time for another pill.

{9}

THE DOCTOR IS IN (ALAS!)

• • •

Good resolutions are useless attempts
to interfere with scientific law.

OSCAR WILDE

Razors pain you;
Rivers are damp;
Acid stains you:
And drugs cause cramp.
Guns aren't lawful;
Nooses give;
Gas smells awful;
You might as well live.

DOROTHY PARKER

Good news for any guy who has read this far (or had this book read to him to this point): this book has now paid for itself by informing you of the things every man needs to know to live longer and healthier, and doubtless, millions of you have determined to institute a new and better lifestyle, with regular prostate exams, routine testicular self-examination, a much healthier diet, and lots and lots of exercise. And although most of you are probably willing to start doing the testicular self-exam part this minute (maybe some of you are even doing it as you read along, but hey, I don't want to know, OK?), as a cynical realist, I also know that most of you are not nearly as willing to start doing the exercise and healthy eating parts, and you're probably particularly willing to forego the prostate exams and colon cancer screening for at least a few days (perhaps many months), because today it's just too (take your pick) late, early, hot, cold, dry, wet, balmy, or windy, and you're just too tired, alive, scared, exuberant, anxious, and so on, to do anything but read some more of this rivetting book. After all, tomorrow is another day, isn't it? (Which reminds me, isn't *Annie* the smarmiest musical you ever had to sit through? Aside from *Cats* and that interminable *Phantom*, of course.)

So despite my pleading and exhortations, I know very well that only a small handful of you will actually do even a bit of what I have advised you to do. And even those of you who do set off tomorrow to live a healthier life will nearly all soon abandon your efforts and will instead pick one of the readily available excuses that come in a handy boxed set at Wal-Mart (my wife's bookstore is willing to match Wal-Mart's price, by the way)—you're too old, it's too hard, there's not enough time, you're allergic to exercise, you don't have the right clothes, you don't want to outlive your kids—to wave at anyone, especially your wife, who tries to get you to do some of the things we discussed in this book.

Rather than dealing with the inevitable health valleys that await you, most of you, I predict, will begin relying on doctors to get you through. Most middle-aged men, you see, seem to labour under the delusion that all they have to do to keep their health together or to reassemble it when it breaks down temporarily (they hope) is to 1) get an annual physical examination and some tests, which will undoubtedly detect the few potentially life-threatening diseases they are prone to at a stage when those problems are still treatable, and 2) get some medications to fix whatever abnormalities are detected. As if. If only.

An Annual Physical Examination Is about as Valuable as an Opinion from Paris Hilton

I hate to prick your balloon, guys, but annual physical examinations for middle-aged gents are vastly overrated. By overrated I don't mean to imply that men especially like to have an annual physical. ("You really ought to visit this new doctor I've just been to. Man, when this guy tells you to turn your head and cough, it's heaven. Why are you looking at me like that, Norm?") Rather, it's that men tend to think that getting a regular annual physical is a valuable insurance policy against sudden death. They may get sick, they think, but they surely won't die all of a sudden if the doctor evaluates them regularly and picks up the earliest signs of a wonky ticker or a lump in their nether parts.

Wrong. Wrong. Wrong. Although getting an annual full physical examination that turns out to be normal will no doubt lower your anxiety level and help you sleep better (it will certainly help your doctor sleep better, given the fees the doctor earns for doing a physical), there is absolutely no proof that in healthy individuals annual complete physical exams detect important hidden medical problems or, more important, that they actually save lives. Why? Because during midlife, I'm afraid, most of us get symptoms when we get sick, and in a middle-aged man, it's rare for a routine physical exam to detect a cancer or a metabolic abnormality, for example, before the disease has betrayed its presence with symptoms that the patient ought to have noticed. Ought to have noticed, I stress, because the majority of men ignore obvious physical symptoms for as long as possible.

That is not to say that doctors don't detect abnormalities when they do routine physicals. They do indeed come across lots of them, too many, in fact, because most of the abnormalities they find are of no real importance as harbingers of life-limiting disease, and you really don't need to know about them. Once an abnormality is picked up, however, the doctor often feels obligated, from the sudden anxiety evident in the patient's demeanour, to do some tests "just to be sure" there's nothing wrong. ("I think we should do a CT scan, George, just to be sure this is a real paper cut." "And maybe an MRI, too, doc? I don't mind the wait." "Sure, George.") This is often bad medicine because not only can tests yield false-positive results (see below), but medical tests also invariably produce at least some degree of anxiety until the results are in, not to mention that every test also carries a small degree of risk—even a blood test can result in a blood clot or an infection.

A false-positive result is one that indicates the presence of an abnormality when in fact everything's OK. The problem with false-positives is that they often require more testing with procedures such as biopsies, for example, that are not only invasive but that carry their own risks, not to mention the consequent anxiety until those latter results are in.

Bottom line: you really don't want unnecessary tests. And you certainly never want, as so many men request, "to be tested for everything." That road leads to chaos.

So the next time you're tempted to go for a physical examination even though your health has been excellent, just remember this old homily you can needlepoint onto something to hang on your bedroom wall: the more doctors poke, the more they find. The more they find, the more they test. The more they test, the more they find. The more they find, the more they test, and on and on, sort of like Ravel's *Bolero.*

In all fairness, I must point out that my opinion about the lack of benefits from routine physicals is a minority one among my colleagues. Thus, a recent study found that although many family docs recognize and acknowledge the aforementioned limits to and drawbacks inherent in annual physical exams, a majority still believe in the overall value of annual exams, mostly because, they say, the routine exam serves as an excellent vehicle to get often reluctant patients (read: men) into the office, and because routine exams also foster much better doctor-patient communication. You're more likely, these doctors aver, to discuss your marriage problems with a doctor who has gone over you a few times with you in your briefs (and less) than to do so with a doctor you've only seen for the briefest few moments when you had some sort of rash or sore throat.

And lest you think that it's only older, more cynical male docs who think that way, this survey concluded that it was actually younger, female doctors who were most in favour of routine annual physicals. I don't agree with this reasoning, which I think is pretty self-serving, but then, what's new in that, eh?

Having pooh-poohed the benefit of annual physical exams for most men, I do not want to give you the idea that all routine visits to your doctor are a waste of time. On the contrary, some routine exams are vital. Most important, those men who have health problems or who have particular health risks—if you have a family history of premature death from heart disease, for example, or if you have had an abnormal blood glucose test (see Chapter 5)—should definitely get regular checkups. What that means is that your special risks and the state of your health—not the inviolate calendar—should determine how often and for which conditions you need to be routinely examined.

And even if you have no health risks, all of you should still have some partial exams regularly.

- You should have your blood pressure checked routinely, probably once a year, although for the average-risk or low-risk male, I believe that can be safely done by one of those shopping-centre blood-pressure reading machines that are pretty accurate screening gauges of blood pressure. However, if you visit the doctor for any other reason, why not have her take your blood pressure once a year, too?
- You might also want to have your prostate palpated regularly. Perhaps I should rephrase that and say that you should have your prostate palpated regularly—probably once a year—whether you want to or not. I can't actually prove to you that all that handling of your prostate will make a difference in your health outcome, but it's one of those things that doctors seem married to, and I just can't go against the grain on this one.

The need for other regular exams is much more debatable. Some people believe you should get your skin examined for skin cancer regularly—and that's by a doctor, please note, not by your significant other, although getting the latter to do it is clearly likely to be a lot more fun than getting lab-coated Dr. S. to go over you. Again, it probably doesn't matter much to the average-risk person, but this examination is very important if you are at high risk for skin cancer, and particularly for malignant melanoma. This includes anyone who has had lots of sun exposure or previous skin cancers, has fair skin, has lots of moles, is redheaded, or has a history of bad sunburns in childhood and adolescence.

Another debatable recommendation is to get regular eye examinations with an emphasis on screening for glaucoma, as well as conditions such as cataracts and age-related macular degeneration. Again, I would certainly comply if I were in a high-risk category for glaucoma (people of African descent, for example), but I am just not convinced of the need to do regular screening for such conditions in the average-risk population. That said, I love spending time with my ophthalmologist (his eye charts are just so cute!), so I often go see him just for the heck of it.

You should also get some medical tests on a regular basis, although unfortunately, routine screening has turned into a political minefield. Some of these tests are not covered by some medical plans and you may need to reach into your own wallet to pay for them:

- As a healthy midlife man, you should get your cholesterol profile (see Chapter 5) done at least once, and depending on the readings and your lifestyle and risk factors, you should get it rechecked periodically until well into your porch-sitting years (oh, about fifty-four, or so).
- You should get a blood glucose reading regularly starting at about age forty-five (see Chapter 5), and at a younger age if you have a strong family history of Type II diabetes or if you're significantly overweight.
- You should not back away from getting regular tests for colorectal cancer (see Chapter 5).
- You should also at least think about the PSA test (Chapter 4) and decide whether you believe that screening is a good idea given the current limitations with that test, or whether this is a test that you can delay until they refine it a bit more.

One thing, though: no matter which of the foregoing tests and examinations you decide to get and which you decide to omit, for heaven's sake, remember the results, especially any numerical readings. As I wrote earlier, one man's "high" is another man's "mellow," so informing a worried new doctor you're seeing for the first time that you were recently told that your blood pressure is slightly high is about as useful to him as providing a partial home phone number for Jennifer Garner—it's a start but it won't really get him—or you—anywhere.

One final piece of advice: keep your immunizations up-to-date. This includes routine tetanus-diphtheria boosters, as well as boosters for other immunizations you might require such as for pneumonia. As to other vaccines, this is an ever-changing landscape, and a matter of quite some debate even among the experts (SARS and avian flu, anyone?), but among the shots you are likely to have to consider over the next few years, you can include:

- pneumonia (depends on your age and your risk factors, but I'd get this one if I were at risk; actually, I am and I did)
- hepatitis A (I'd advise getting this one, too, especially if you travel lots; I do and I did)
- hepatitis B (ditto, but this one also depends a lot on the risks you take when you travel, or at home, for that matter; I got this one, too—well, you just never know, do you? I mean, of course, you never know when you might need a blood transfusion overseas. What did you think I meant?)
- chicken pox (if you're at risk)
- mumps-measles-rubella (again, depending on risk)
- special vaccines for travel
- whooping cough
- shingles (this one will likely come along very soon, and it makes sense to me)

And don't forget to at least consider getting an annual flu shot (I get one every autumn, but then, I hate getting sick and no one pays me if I'm off work).

"Be Careful about Reading Health Books. You Might Die of a Misprint"—Mark Twain

Many midlife men, after a youth spent avoiding a doctor's visit for as long as possible, begin to visit the doctor whenever they feel ill or develop even the slightest new symptom. This happens, unfortunately, because midlife is when most men begin to see death's visage staring back at them in every itch or cough or red blotch that pops up. This is when a wife becomes indispensable, by the way, because a wife is the one person who will invariably say the only words you really need to hear during these panic attacks: "Grow up, Frank."

If a wife doesn't deflect your urge to sit in the doctor's office 24/7, though, let me warn you about beginning to rely on your doctor to alleviate your concerns about every new symptom. The doctor is not a magician. She does not have other-world diagnostic skills to determine what's bothering you (one study has estimated that nearly 50 per cent of visits to the doctor end without a diagnosis that can be confirmed; but then that's why they call it medical practice, I think), and she doesn't possess a grab bag of miracle potions to make you feel better. You may have misplaced it over the years, but most of you were born with a modicum of good sense. Find it and use it. Instead of your doctor, rely more on the well-tested remedy of "tincture of time," or the advice and counsel of your significant other, and you'll probably do just as well, often even better.

Unfortunately, there is no cut-and-dried set of rules to tell you when a visit to the doctor is necessary, and everyone has a story about a Poor Joe. "Didn't see the doctor with his four-day cough and now he has double pneumonia." (In my mother's world, no one ever gets "single pneumonia," but invariably two pneumonias for the price of one cold.) We all feel sorry for Poor Joe, of course, but the truth is that it's very unlikely Poor Joe's doctor could have prevented his pneumonia even if Poor Joe had been sitting in the doctor's office all during his illness. "But," some of you are no doubt sputtering, "even if it doesn't do us any good to see the doctor quickly with our symptoms, surely it can't do us any harm." Poor naïve babies. First, think back to that old needlepoint homily from a few paragraphs ago. Also, the more you visit the doctor, the more likely you are to get a prescription for some kind of medication, and the unwarranted use of drugs in many situations has become a major source of medical harm (see below).

Even more important, doctors make mistakes. A Harris poll in the U.S. found that 42 per cent of respondents claim that they or a friend or a relative have experienced a "medical mistake." Fortunately, most of those errors were probably minor and didn't involve loss of life (although I am not sure how they would have gone about trying to poll those who were actually killed by medical mistakes), but even minor errors can be uncomfortable or lead to further problems.

Another practice that's become much more common (and problematic) in midlife is to start consulting the Internet for every new twitch, twinge, and tic. The Internet, however, is the ultimate mixed blessing. So while often offering excellent information and advice, much of what you get on the Internet comes with very little perspective (actually, none), and as often as it delivers a valuable answer for a specific question, the Internet can and does lead to many worrisome and sleepless nights by overstating the potential consequences of a symptom or occurrence. This is especially the case in disease-oriented chat rooms where many of the visitors have been driven by the need to tell their story of medical mishandling, which is, however, as often as not, a one-off rather than the norm. The Internet can be an invaluable assistant in investigating unusual complaints and new therapies, and depending on the Web site, the Internet also offers excellent and up-to-date overviews of medical problems and conditions. As with everything, use your common sense.

If You Do Visit the Doctor, Be a Kid and Ask Why, Why, Why

I think many of you would gain a lot by becoming more like many of my old patients. No, I don't mean you have to turn into an ex-hippy who now drives a Volvo station wagon instead of a painted-on Beetle and who is more interested in thanking you with dope on stock tips than with plain old regular dope (never took the stock tips, by the way). Rather, what I mean is that you need to be a lot more assertive and skeptical in your doctor's office. Thus, when you visit your family doc, always make sure to:

- Bring along useful information such as a list of your pills and natural remedies, and even a family history record. (For most men, the most useful source of information, of course, is a voluble wife who can accompany her slower-witted husband on his visit.)
- Be specific and concise about what brought you into the office. ("Nancy thought I had something but I'm not really sure what she was talking about" is not going to get you very far with the average family doctor who, studies show, interrupts the patient within thirty seconds of the start of an office visit, although to be frank, I don't know how most of my colleagues hold on even that long.)
- Have a clear timeline of symptoms ready to tell the busy physician. ("I'm not sure how long my tongue has been blue" is not going to get you the best service.)
- Be honest about what you have—and haven't—done for yourself. (On a followup visit, for example, fess up if you really haven't taken the pills the doctor told you on the previous visit were the sole solution to your problem. And likewise, if you've put your faith in a vial of strange-smelling liquid your Croatian cleaning lady assured you was what all the peasants back home used when they had what you have and now you're feeling much worse, hey, be honest enough to mention that, too.)

- Most important: ask lots of questions and always challenge your doctor to answer your concerns.

So when you leave a doctor's office, the bare minimum you should know is the answer to these questions:

- What do I have? (Oh, it's a virus.)
- What else could it be? (You don't think it's Ebola? I know I haven't been to Africa, but I did go to the zoo once when I was a kid.)
- When should I expect to be better? (Should I tell my boss I won't be back till 2009? [For unionized workers, 2019.])
- What should I do if I am not better in that time? (What if I get the Marburg virus and avian flu on top of this?)
- What can I do to make myself better? (Rest at home? Have more sex? Want to tell my wife that?)
- Should I contact you again? (Why are you sneering, doc?)

If you receive a prescription, here are a few more questions you need to have answered:

- What is this drug? (this is particularly important to ask when you get a free sample from the bottom of the doctor's desk, especially if the sample is covered with dust and is stamped "Best used before Oct 1912")
- Why this drug and not another? (You know, doc, my brother-in-law has exactly the same thing and his doctor gave him a blue pill, not a red one. You sure I need this red one?)
- How safe is it? (This is not another Vioxx [see below] like you gave me a few months back, eh, doc? Just kidding. I'm still here, and lucky for you, too.)
- Are there any alternative medications?
- How do I take it? (Four times a day? Does that also include weekends?)
- Anything I should avoid while I'm on it? (Is it OK to take this with my nightly cocktail? Which one?)
- Anything it interacts with? (This doesn't interfere with Viagra, does it, doc? No, you never prescribed Viagra for me and I'm not getting it off the net. I'm just curious, that's all.)

If you are sent for tests, here are some other questions you need to have answered:

- Why do I need this test?
- Could the results of this test change what we plan on doing anyway?

- Is it safe—what are the risks?
- How accurate is this test at detecting what we want to find?
- When will you have the results?
- Can I get the results over the phone?

This last point raises a pet peeve of mine. With certain exceptions—the HIV test being the most obvious example—I believe that most test results can be given over the phone, although for various reasons related to fees, the pressure on office staff, and concern about how the patient will take the result, many doctors prefer to give test results in a face-to-face meeting. Since most test results are normal, however, it seems to me to be an unbelievable waste of time, effort, and money to have someone come back to the office to hear that "your cholesterol level [or throat culture or Pap smear] was normal. Next."

Bottom line: when you leave a doctor's office, you should possess a very clear idea of what you have, what's likely to happen to you, and why you are treating it or investigating it in the manner you've agreed to. This will not only spare you lots of hassle on the home front (you know damn well that you'll be subjected to an inquisition when you get home, and "I didn't ask" is going to get you the absolute worst punishment that can be meted out) but it will also save you a lot of anxiety ("Did he say 'Ebola' or 'granola'? Think harder.")

Now on first thought, you might expect that the answers to all the questions I listed would take the doctor about a year to dispense. As a long-time family physician, however, I can tell you that most of us have learned to speak so fast that we go through this checklist in only a few minutes, especially if you don't interrupt our stream of words, and those few minutes are a good investment in preventing needless extra visits to the office.

When It Comes to Drugs, Just Say No (More Often)

We live in a culture and an era that demands chemical answers for every symptom or illness—a pill for every ill, "a med for my head else I'm dead"—and too many doctors are only too keen to feed our habit. Thus, a whopping 44 per cent of American adults take at least one prescription drug daily, while 17 per cent take three or more, and please note that this doesn't include over-the-counter drugs, which are also very heavily used. Happily, most of the time the medications you get from your doctor or take on your own are helpful and don't lead to (too many) side effects and adverse reactions. But as that Harris poll I referred to earlier also found, at least 28 per cent of patients claim they know that they have been subjected to a drug error, and if you factor in all those patients who have no clue that the drug they were taking is what caused their hair to turn green or their feet to smell like ripe cheese (more than usually, that is), that rate of health problems associated with the use of medications is probably much higher.

There are many ways to be adversely affected by drugs. For a start, there are the common side effects associated with all drugs, synthetic and natural (even herbal products produce side effects, something most natural product advocates want you to ignore). Most side effects are merely nuisance symptoms—nausea, headaches, upset stomach, gas—but even those relatively minor adjustments can make life quite unpleasant, not just for the person who gets the symptoms but also for those forced to deal with the nauseous, headachey, burping and farting pill-taker. Although side effects often occur at normal doses of a drug, they tend to become more common with higher doses.

Another way to be adversely affected by medication is to receive the wrong medication for your condition, or to get the wrong dose of medication. Fortunately, this doesn't occur often, but it does happen more than we care to admit. So when someone is asking you to take a pill, for example, in hospital, always ask some questions before swallowing: "Is this the medication I've been prescribed? What's it called, by the way? And what's the dose?" I know this will upset some of your health care providers, but honestly, would you rather suffer a convulsion or have a nurse angry with you?

But the secret you may not know is that you don't have to take the wrong drug to be harmed by medication: even the right drug at the proper dose can harm you, what is referred to in medical parlance as an "adverse drug reaction" (ADR). Adverse drug reactions stem from the *proper* use of drugs—no mistakes were made when the drugs were used, and the drugs were only doing what they were supposed to do but something untoward happened anyway. Adverse drug reactions most often occur because of:

- interaction with another drug or drugs or even with something else the patient is ingesting (for example, grapefruit juice contains an enzyme that interacts with lots of drugs, including high blood pressure medications, cardiac medications, statins, some hormones, anti-allergy drugs, even Viagra and Cialis, so never, Big Guy, gulp your Viagra with a grapefruit juice chaser)
- an exaggerated response in an individual to a normal dose of a drug
- an allergic or idiosyncratic reaction to a specific drug

Unfortunately, adverse drug reactions are very common and account for thousands of complications and deaths yearly (one very hyped and controversial study concluded that ADRS are the sixth leading cause of death in North America). And occasionally we don't learn about certain adverse reactions—or take them seriously enough—until a drug has been on the market for a while, sometimes even years. That's what happened in the case of the COX-2 inhibitor, rofecoxib (Vioxx). Although studies first raised awareness of the potential cardiovascular risk associated with Vioxx as early as 1999, it wasn't until five years later that the drug was finally withdrawn from the market because of the evidence that some people who took Vioxx suffered heart attacks as a direct consequence of taking that drug. Bottom line: don't take medications—vitamins, herbs, or manufactured drugs—if you don't need to. You just never know.

But if they can be so dangerous, why do doctors give out so many drugs, even in situations where it's unclear if a drug is warranted? Several reasons. First, for most of you, there's that very firmly expressed wish to take drugs whenever you're ill. Quite simply, too many of you clearly want drugs when you see your doctor, and it's far easier for a doctor to give you what you want than it is to spend the extra time and effort convincing you that medication is not the answer to your problem. Thus, studies show that patients who expect a drug are between three and ten times more likely to get one as those who don't expect to be medicated by the doctor.

Then, there's us doctors, who are only too happy to supply your wishes because we're here to help you, and generally the potentially quickest way to do that comes via a salve or a pill or a potion, not to ignore the fact that in this litigious era of malpractice suits, it seems much safer to give something, anything, even if the condition doesn't warrant it than it is to say, "Hey, let's just do nothing and see what happens."

Finally, there's the two of us, the combination of doctors and patients, who have been programmed to believe that drugs do far more good than the objective evidence often indicates. So for a variety of reasons, not the least of which is the unbelievable amount of pro-medication advertising generated by pharmaceutical companies, doctors and the public generally tend to ignore the potential harmful consequences of medication while focussing primarily on the benefits. (Big letters: "This amazing drug can get rid of zits. Just ask your doctor." Tiny, tiny letters: "This drug can cause headaches, strokes, and a loss of interest in sex.") Hey, take the pimples, man. And if you do decide to treat the zits, read the fine print in those drug ads—those side effects do happen to people like you. Also, remember that if you do get any new symptoms while taking a drug, it might be because of the drug, so call your doctor or pharmacist and ask about that possibility.

Are there some drugs that are more overused than others? Of course. Although studies (and prejudices) vary in pointing fingers, for me, antibiotics, nonsteroidal anti-inflammatories (NSAIDS, see Chapter 5), and antidepressants (see Chapter 8) are especially likely to be overprescribed.

There is no dispute about this: many antibiotic prescriptions are unnecessary, especially those dispensed for upper respiratory infections, which are most often caused by viruses and thus are not amenable to the usual battery of bug killers. Yes, we do have some anti-viral drugs but these have very specific indications and uses, and thank god, these drugs are still not being overprescribed in North America, although as always, that's not the case in Asia, where they are being prescribed freely, which means they may not work over here when and if they're finally needed (for example, to help contain a flu pandemic).

But antibiotics (for bacteria) are still being way overprescribed by North American doctors, despite all the attention paid to this issue in medical journals and continuing medical education courses. So although doctors have gotten better at putting the brakes on antibiotic use than they were years ago for certain conditions (ear infections in kids, for example, for which antibiotic use has dropped quite significantly), doctors are not doing nearly as good a job at halting unnecessary antibiotic use in other conditions, most prominently upper respiratory infections. Thus, a headline over an editorial from the mid-nineties in an eminent journal, the *Lancet,* asked "What will it take to stop physicians from prescribing antibiotics in acute bronchitis?" Yet a followup study in 2004 found that most doctors were still prescribing antibiotics for "acute bronchitis," even though we all know that the vast majority of bronchitis infections are caused by viruses and even though there is no evidence at all that using antibiotics for bronchitis will either cut the duration of a bronchitis infection, lessen the symptoms of cough and phlegm production, reduce the time you spend coughing, or prevent bronchitis from going on to become pneumonia, should the infection decide to move down into your lungs. In other words, the drugs don't work and they don't protect, yet they are still being dispensed. (As an important aside: a recent study showed that the average upper respiratory infection produced a cough that lasted—on average, mind—twenty-one days, and that the cough in over one-quarter of such infections lasts twenty-eight days. And these infections are not ameliorated in any way through the use of antibiotics.)

But what's wrong with getting an antibiotic the next time you cough up a little bit too much phlegm or want to make sure you don't get sicker because you're flying off to Hawaii to compete in the Iron Man Potato Sack Run? Lots.

First, there's the nuisance of side effects, which can be pretty severe on some antibiotics. I don't know about you, but taking a drug that I don't need that then gives me diarrhea, gas, and a headache is a joy I can live without.

Second, there's the risk of complications. Antibiotics don't just kill the harmful bugs. They kill lots of useful bugs, too, some of which are actually keeping other nasty critters out of your system. For example, a nasty bug known as *Clostridium difficile* has become a huge problem in patients who enter Quebec-area hospitals, as well as in the UK, largely because of the overuse of antibiotics. Another recent study showed that the common remedy of using antibiotics for as little as six weeks to treat acne doubles a person's risk of developing an upper respiratory infection, probably because the antibiotic interferes with the normal bacteria that help repel many of these viral critters that are always trying to infect us.

Perhaps most seriously, though, the more antibiotics we give out, the faster those potentially dangerous little bacteria that lurk everywhere may develop resistance to them, so that those overused antibiotics will be useless when we really need them.

Bottom line: don't use antibiotics when you don't have to. And remember especially that even a diagnosis of "bronchitis" generally doesn't mean you need antibiotics.

As for NSAIDS, besides the warnings you read about in Chapter 5 such as a higher risk of ulcers and bleeding from the stomach associated with the use of these drugs, be aware that when NSAIDS are used to treat headaches, they produce an effect known as rebound in which a chronic user of analgesics gets a bad headache when he temporarily tries to stop his use of those drugs, prompting him—naturally—to take even more of the drugs.

If, after considering this information, you do decide you need to use medication to treat a particular problem, here are a few other cautions to take heed of. First, always take the smallest dose of the weakest medication for the least amount of time that will do the trick, because the higher the dose, the more likely you are to run into those unwanted effects discussed earlier. And you might question your doctor about this one, too, because most prescriptions are written with an average large male in mind, and many people, such as this small male author, to be sure, can get the same effect from many drugs by cutting the dose in half, or even in quarters. Besides, we all differ in our response to medications. Sleeping pills are an excellent example. I can generally nod off on one-quarter of the pill I prefer (zoplicone, if you must know), while my wife just has to look at one to get the same effect. On the other hand, some people need the full dose to get to sleep.

Also, and I know this may sound like your mother (but then what's wrong with that, Mr. Big Shot?), remember that a drug only works if you take it. Sit up straight, by the way. And wipe that smile off your face, midlife man. You can't fool me, because studies show that 50 per cent of prescription drugs are not taken as directed and that 20 per cent are never taken at all. So, listen up, Mr. Never-Does-Anything-Like-He-Was-Told-To-Do-It. If you want to get your cholesterol levels down, the cholesterol-lowering medication won't work if it stays in your medicine cabinet. You may want to argue about the dose, but if your cholesterol levels are high, you really want to take at least some of the drug you've been put on.

Can you stop taking a drug before the prescription runs out? Depends. With some drugs, particularly, antibiotics, you should always finish the full prescription (so long as the prescription was warranted to begin with, of course). With other drugs, you can prematurely discontinue them if the condition improves, or if your situation changes, although you should always discuss this option with your doctor before stopping any medication cold.

{10}

HAPPINESS AND HEALTH COME IN MANY WAYS

• • •

Health is a state of complete physical,
mental and social well-being, not merely the
absence of disease or infirmity.

CONSTITUTION OF THE WORLD HEALTH ORGANIZATION

It's not that I'm afraid to die.
I just don't want to be there when it happens.

WOODY ALLEN, *Death (A Play)*

So, that's it, guys: all you really need to know about what you are going through or are about to go through, and most important, what you can still do to make your last few (sorry about that) years happier and healthier. Sadly, however, no matter how diligent you are at following my sage advice, I'm afraid that you are still not going to live forever. So even if you never smoke another cigarette, cigar, or poorly rolled, funny-smelling thingie handed you at a boring party by a bearded, scruffy, tweed coated, nonsense-spouting, self-absorbed bigmouth who turns out to be the guy teaching your kids at university; even if you scrupulously minimize your exposure to all toxins, even so far as to avoid sitting on leather couches just to be 100 per cent certain that you don't come down with mad cow disease; even if you have a great social support system as a result of working hard at being a good spouse and worker and parent and the most valuable member of your competitive drinking team; even if you never go out without a hat on and without slathering on the sunscreen, even on a cloudy day in December; even if you practise safe sex when you're alone because, hey, these days you never can tell; even if you eat tons of health-promoting veggies (keeping in mind that a veg prepared in the British fashion, that is, boiled and blanched and then stored for three weeks before being reheated in the microwave and left for an hour before being served, is not a veg—I'm not sure what it is, but vegetable it is not); even if you regularly run half-marathons mostly because you love to watch the latex-garbed ladies run by you; even if you meditate so often that OM has now become your nickname at the kabala house of worship you now attend on a regular basis to help you locate your true inner self; even if you become such a good guy that it now takes you twenty minutes to dress every day because of all the wrist bands and ribbons you have to put on to let the world know which causes you support, you may still be doomed to an earlier death or more chronic diseases than that lazy, friendless, obese sloth next door whose daily fare consists of two deep-fried Mars bar, several hot dogs, and many bags of chips, who sics his Doberman on anyone who comes to his trailer door seeking money to support either the rebels in Bantustan or Greenpeace, and who never moves his butt except to waddle to the car to buy more smokes and beer.

As my wife often laments after some item in the news has caught her attention, "There really is no justice," and that's particularly so, I submit, when it comes to health and well-being, because much of what happens to us is a product of our uncontrollable (at least up to this point) early environment and genes.

C'est simply la vie, I'm afraid. For example, several studies of centenarians found that the best chance you have of living to a hundred is directly related to whether your parent or sibling (or better yet, parents and siblings) also lived to a hundred. Another study on the benefits of having a high HDL cholesterol level found that the best determinant of high HDL was (ta dum) having parents with high HDL levels. Whatever it is that your parents gave you, you're stuck with that, I'm afraid.

Happily, you can modify at least some of the effects your genes exert, and that's what you should always aim to do—work on those lifestyle factors that are known to influence health and well-being, especially the ones that you feel are worth working on.

When you've had enough of doing that, however, it's equally important to lean back, stop feeling guilty about what you have still not gotten around to doing and may in fact never get around to, and relax and enjoy these best years of your life before the next stage of your all-too-brief sojourn in this mortal realm. Maximizing happiness is, after all, what it's all about.

And that clearly doesn't necessarily come only via proper diet and exercise and not smoking. No, even the medical literature shows that there are many, many, many non-lifestyle doors to happiness, and happily for you, I am quite prepared to be your guide to some of those portals of pleasure, to be your good times guru, your sunshine swami, your happiness harpy, and the only charge I levy is the price of this book (no charge, of course, if you borrowed it from the library, but only if you get it back in time). Here, then, are some suggestions not related to lifestyle that can make you either happier or improve your life expectancy, perhaps even both.

Improve Your Sex Life

I start with this because lots of men believe fervently that one of the keys to greater happiness is a better sex life. In fact, I'm sure it's the unstated promise that reading this book will surely improve their sex lives that got a lot of guys to even pick it up in the first place. So for those guys who want to increase their happiness quotient by improving their sex lives, learning what turns women on and what makes women happier, and then adopting appropriate tactics, here are some often-overlooked observations and strategies that just might help you.

1. Make More Money

Not only do studies show that the rich have more sex than those of us of lesser means (so just imagine what Bill Gates's or Warren Buffet's love lives must be like; better yet, don't), but a survey also found that women worry more about money than do men, and that women are more likely to think about money than sex—no surprise to most men, of course, although it may surprise some women that there are also some men who think about money more than sex. What's wrong with those guys, anyway? Bottom line: just get her mind off the bucks and she's bound to focus on the buck instead, right?

2. Take Her Shopping More Often

If you want to give your partner multiple orgasms, and who doesn't, as long as it doesn't take all night, of course, you should know that a survey for the Factory Outlet Marketing Association found that 46 per cent of women would rather find a great bargain on clothes than have great sex. So why not take her to Saks or Holt Renfrew, and then try to sneak into the change room with her? Only make sure it's the right change room.

3. Give Her More to Do

According to Dr. Jean Claude Kaufmann, a sociologist from the Sorbonne in Paris, where they are said to know a thing or two about matters of love and sex, housewives find that activities such as vacuuming and dusting induce "heightened emotions of love or hate" and that repeated participation in these activities leads to feelings that are akin to those experienced from erotic love. As a househusband of many years' standing, though, I have to say that this is either one of those French things that we just can't relate to (such as eating eels and snails, or smoking Gitanes) or more likely it's one of those women things men can't relate to. I mean, when I'm home alone all day, I keep staring at that ironing board, but it's never done anything for me. The Cuisinart, on the other hand...

4. Get Her Lots of Chocolate

You won't be surprised to learn, I'm sure, that a survey done, not coincidentally, for the Confectionery Manufacturers Association, found that 38 per cent of Canadian women prefer chocolate to more sex, although you may be surprised to learn that 30 per cent of Canadian men made the same choice. Speaking only for myself, I like both, but it can get really messy.

5. Get Yourself Fixed

According to a survey done for Marie Stopes International, a British family planning charity, vasectomy is quick and painless and can improve your sex life. In fact, it's so pleasant, the survey found, that 92 per cent of men said they would recommend it to a friend. I agree. I recommend vasectomies to all my friends, and one day I might even be brave enough to find out what one is really like. Actually, Marie Stopes International is so convinced that more men would get vasectomies if they only knew how safe and easy they are, they've now posted a real-time video on the net in which you can see an actual vasectomy being performed, although I, for one, think this tactic will likely backfire big-time and that most men who view this video will talk themselves out of going for the operation. Why? Because any guy watching that film will, without doubt, see the thin surgical blade the surgeon is shown using as more like a cleaver or machete.

6. Get a Personality

When *Psychology Today* readers were asked to rank the important features that would attract them to a man, I was blown away by how well I did, so let's see how you stack up, guys. Women ranked intelligence first (got that), sense of humour second (check), followed by ability to talk about feelings (OK, minus that), ability to empathize (minus that one, too, so back to square one), facial appearance (I have facial appearance, but I'm not the best judge of how good it is, so call this one a draw), overall body build (minus four), sexual performance (hey! way back in plus territory), and physical strength (well, for my size, and with my new abs, I'm not too bad there). See? Now you know what women want.

7. Become More Attractive

Besides making yourself more attractive with cosmetic surgery and subterfuge creams, another way to do it is to conceal your less attractive features, that is, to use camouflage in the form of garments that hide the true condition your condition is in, something that lots of men seem to be doing. Among the items men are apparently purchasing in order to look better, there are such ego boosters as Slenderizing Manshape Undergarments, Super Shaper Briefs, and Butt Booster (although honestly, folks, how many straight men do you know who actually need a bigger butt?). If you're ridiculous enough to think you need such items, then go get them, but be forewarned, Big Guy, that my Manshapes were so tight they made my reflux symptoms much worse.

Rather than camouflage, some of you might prefer to concentrate on just becoming more symmetrical because it has been claimed that the most symmetrical faces are rated the most attractive. For example, men with the most symmetrical faces lose their virginity earlier and tend to have more sexual partners than men whose noses are where their ears should be. And a study in the *New Scientist* claims that being symmetrical is better for your partner too. According to this study, if a woman's partner is "very symmetrical," women reach orgasm 75 per cent of the time, while with lopsided partners, they reach orgasm only 30 per cent of the time. That shouldn't be all that surprising, though. After all, common sense tells me that it's harder to reach orgasm when the other person in bed looks like someone straight out of a Picasso painting. I mean, what part would you focus on if you were faced with a Picasso subject? And how would you even know you were being faced?

8. Smell Better

A study from the Smell and Taste Research Foundation in Chicago claims that male sexual arousal can be turned on by the odours of pumpkin pie, donuts, licorice, and lavender, which can then send blood rushing to the penis. I have news for those researchers: there's nothing special about the smell of pumpkins or donuts. The average guy is turned on by any smell at all, even year-old sneakers. And most guys are turned on by the absence of smell, too.

9. Or Maybe Just Smell Worse

A study from the Institute of Urban Ethology in Vienna found that women volunteers claimed that the more attractive a man's face was, the less appealing he smelled. So taking that to its logical conclusion, just try to smell awful, and women will find you irresistible, although I believe that this is a tactic already employed by many men, often those in any slow-moving elevator I'm sharing. And guys, the good news is that if you don't smell bad enough naturally, you can always smell worse artificially by buying yourself some underpants pre-scented with sweat. Yes, the Japanese, the patron saints of useless inventions, have invented underpants laced with artificial sweat containing a synthesized pheromone found in the sweat of the underarm. I've ordered eight pairs.

Before you rush off to smell like a man's used locker, though, let me warn you that using smell to entice women is not as simple as it seems. You see, a study on cockroaches published in the journal *Nature* found that the difference between the male cockroaches on the top of the leftover pile in the kitchen and those on the bottom is usually a result of the scents the cockroaches give off, so if a male gives off too much of a status-lowering scent, he quickly becomes a roach feeding off the crumbs left behind by the more dominant roaches. So why, you may wonder, has evolution allowed a status-lowering scent to persist? Because of female roaches, that's why. It turns out, you see, that some female roaches get turned on by the more vulnerable males. Sound familiar?

10. Go Whole Hog

So putting together everything cited above and elsewhere in this book (see the Chapter 3 discussion of factors influencing rates of sexual intercourse in particular), here's what you can do to increase your chances of having a better sex life:

- Buy as many jazz CDs as you can.
- Get yourself a big gun or, even better, several.
- Buy yourself a trailer.
- Park your trailer next to a Saks or Bloomingdale's store, where your mate can shop to her heart's content.
- Buy her lots of household appliances.
- Stock your trailer with tons of chocolate.
- Rob a bank, but get shot while escaping so that you can seem more vulnerable.

- Get as much plastic surgery as you can afford.
- Improve your mind.
- Get yourself fixed.
- Learn to expose your female side.
- Smell worse.

What is sobering, though, is how many men already have many of those bases covered, and it still hasn't done them any good.

By the way, besides leading to more happiness (potentially), more sex may also lead to some health benefits. Thus, a study of middle-aged Welshmen from the town of Caerphilly and its environs found that the more orgasms a male has over a lifetime, the more likely he is to live longer. Now I realize that at first glance this finding might run counter to my earlier speculations that chasing after too much sex might actually decrease one's life expectancy, but it doesn't really, mainly because who ever said that frequency of orgasms had anything to do with having more sex? Especially for Welshmen. It's dark and lonely in those mines, after all.

Improve Other Aspects of Your Life

So that's it for sex: you now know everything you need to know to make yourself deliriously happy by vastly improving your sex life. If, however, you wake up one day to discover that more and more sex didn't really lead to more and more happiness, here are some other tactics and strategies to try to improve your happiness level.

Get Married

I know you didn't think I'd start with this one, but I had to because it probably trumps all the others. Many studies have shown that married men not only outlive their single counterparts, often by several years, but that the former are also generally much happier than the latter. Why? It may simply be that healthier and happier people tend to get married in the first place. (I mean, the average woman, sizing up her future, is much more likely to consider hitching up with a muscular, robust, ever-smiling oaf than with a gimpy-kneed, myopic, droopy nerd, even though, of course, we all know the nerd will very likely eventually out-earn and probably out-live the oaf, but then, it takes a mature woman to recognize that truth.)

It's more likely, though, that married men do better because marriage has many benefits on health. Thus, marriage is known to lead to lower stress levels (see Chapter 8), marriage improves social contact (you've gotta go out and meet people and even talk to them when you're married because, believe me, there's no choice if you want to stay married), and marriage helps men lead healthier lifestyles, again mostly because we're forced to whether we like it or not. "What do you mean, you're not eating lentils? You don't eat the lentils, you don't get the steak, and I call my mom to come over, too."

And for those cynics—mostly older married men—who say that a married man doesn't really live any longer, he just feels as if he's never going to be allowed to die, the consensus is that marriage does lead to better health for men (interestingly, it doesn't do nearly as much for women, but that's for my next book). For example, a British report concluded that not only do married people live longer, they also suffer lower rates of cancer and heart disease, as well as less stress and mental illness, than do both single people and cohabiters, those who live together but who haven't been dragooned into tying the official knot, although as you would expect, staying in a bad marriage is probably worse for your health than going it solo again. And hey, midlifer, some studies even show that the greatest health benefits from marriage accrue to those of us in middle age.

So if you haven't already done so, get married. And stay married, if at all possible. Just think of marriage as you do porridge: it may not look like the best fare when you look at it directly, but you know it's damn good for you. Besides, by fifty, don't you think it's finally time you got your mother off your back? Let a wife deal with her. She will know how to do it better and with less stress.

Get a Pet

Pets are wonderful for your health. Studies have shown that pet owners have lower blood pressures and lower cholesterol levels than people who don't own pets, they visit the doctor less often (a doctor's visit means less time with Precious, after all), they tend to report less stress (until they have to put poor little Roverkins in a kennel, of course), and most of all they report being happier (well, Snookums is so nice to come home to, aren't you Snookie-Wookie?). And never underestimate the benefits (both physical and psychological) that you will get from taking Big Ben for his two daily walks. The physical benefits are obvious, but psychological benefits accrue, too, because let me tell you, folks, for reasons that escape me, women never seem to mind approaching a man with a cute dog, which is why I have four dogs, of course. Just kidding. I'm happily married, after all, so I keep fish instead. Hate walking them, though. And haven't managed to teach them too many tricks.

Join a House of Worship (One That Doesn't Require Wearing a Wrist Band)

There's lots of evidence for health benefits from regular church attendance. For example, a review of over two hundred studies about religion concluded that 75 per cent of the studies showed that religious commitment had positive effects on health and only 7 per cent showed that prayer was bad for your health (perhaps because the latter studies inadvertently included lots of hypocrites, closet atheists, and agnostics). The strongest positive effects on health, as one might expect, were on drug use, alcoholism, and depression, but religious commitment also seemed to have positive effects on rates of cancer, high blood pressure, and heart disease.

No one knows, of course, what it is about religious commitment that may exert this positive effect on health, but the experts speculate that regular attendance at places of worship—churches, synagogues, mosques, sports arenas, poker tournaments—can lead to:

- an improved outlook
- higher self-esteem
- a sense of community
- taking better care of yourself because of encouragement from the other members of the religious institution

My own theory is much simpler. I think it's one of two things: either prayer works (what do you think most of those people are praying for anyway?) or God just wants to keep the true believers around longer. He needs the laughs, I guess.

By the way, for you cynics who want the benefits of religion without the effort involved in being religious, I'm afraid that you actually have to be a committed believer to get those positive effects—one of these studies concluded that those people who only pray at home (sure, sure) actually have overall worse health outcomes than the non-religious.

Even if religion works, though, the problem for most of us is that it's not as easy to get religion as you may think because our ability to believe may actually be governed by our genes. Thus, some researchers are claiming that they've found a sort of "God-spot" in the brain, an area that, they say, governs an innate belief in God. So it may just be that holy rollers are born not made and that true believers are simply those people who have more cells or more activity in the God-spot of their cortex than the rest of us have. Why would anyone have ended up with a large God-spot in the brain, you ask? These researchers claim that an area like that may have evolved over the eons because being religious adds stability to life and hence to society, although I figure it's probably just because God programmed it that way. Amen. Talk about intelligent design! She must be brilliant, although I have to admit to one problem about intelligent design that I can't get beyond: if there really is an intelligent designer who designed this world, why do we have politicians? Or Geraldo?

If You Won't Join a Church, Join Something Else

We clearly evolved to spend lots of time with others (after all, the more of us there are on the savanna, the less chance each of us has of being the one chosen for dinner). So it's no surprise, I guess, that a report in the *Psychological Bulletin* claims that belonging to anything improves both physical and mental health, although I must caution you that it's very unlikely that joining the drink-until-you-puke brotherhood at your local pub was what these researchers had in mind.

If You Won't Join Anything, At Least Get a Friend to Go to Bingo with You

We all very much need social support systems. A recent ten-year-long study from Australia found that seniors who had strong social support systems and many friends had a 22 per cent reduced risk of dying over that decade compared with seniors who had few friends, which was a much greater benefit than was obtained by even having a very close family. This finding—that friends help much more than family—surprised the authors, but it doesn't surprise me in the slightest. After all, your friends will never come after your estate, your friends will never use your computer to visit Web sites that you're ashamed to look at (at least with your wife in the room), your friends will never borrow your car and bring it home three days later ("Sorry, Dad, I forgot that you work.") with a new dent and no gas in the tank, your friends will never empty your wallet and leave you supremely embarrassed when you can't pay for the take-out pizzas you ordered, and best of all, your friends are very unlikely to ever tell you what they really think of you—if, that is, they want to stay your friends. Your family, on the other hand...

Become Dour and Dependable

A sixty-year-long study of a thousand people found that those who were conscientious as kids were 30 per cent less likely to die in any given year than were their more carefree peers. The same study also found that being cheerful in youth was correlated with a 6 per cent increased likelihood of dying in any given year. "Is that," you ask, "because the world really does suck?" Of course not. It's just that the terminally cheerful have a much higher rate of being strangled to death by a close friend than do those who see the world the way it really is.

But what could account for dependable stay-at-home types living longer? A leading investigator concluded that it's probably because "squares" lead well-balanced, well-integrated lives. They are rarely diagnosed with a psychiatric ailment (and that's a good thing because being a square is punishment enough, I think); they rarely abuse alcohol ("No, thank you. Tried it once, didn't like it."); they never use tranquillizers ("No, thank you. Tried it once, didn't like it."); and they also, of course, have only one child each, sometimes none, depending on whether their partners used birth control on that single occasion.

If You Can't Become Dour, Become More Optimistic

A six-year-long Finnish study found that middle-aged men who feel hopeless about the future and about their chances of attaining their goals are far more likely to die early from coronary heart disease, accidents, and violent deaths than are equally healthy but more hopeful men, which clearly wouldn't surprise guys who are expecting the worst anyway.

According to another British study, every moment of happiness counts in helping reduce stress hormone levels and the risk of subsequent illness. And most troubling perhaps, another study found that the most pessimistic people had the highest risk of dementia, news that will probably bum most pessimistic people out even more. So stop being so pessimistic and think positively instead. Hey! Your son really will move out one day. Taxes are bound to fall eventually. And you can become the next Pope (this guy is getting on, after all), although some of you may have to convert first. Anything's possible if you believe it.

But remember: you can't just fake optimism and good vibes. According to a British researcher, people who constantly have to pretend to be in a good mood, such as those folks who greet you when you walk into Wal-Mart, are more likely to develop stress-related diseases than other people, due to the constant strain of faking a good mood. So don't have a nice day, OK?

Eat Farmed Salmon, Shoot Bears, and Buy Huge SUVs

A study in *Circulation* found that worries about social conditions correlated most closely with negative effects on the heart. So no more money for

Greenpeace, eh, and let the bloody whales and dolphins save themselves. And the forests and rivers? Hey, let David Suzuki worry about those for you. He's glad to do it for you, I'm sure.

Watch Politicians at Work on CPAC or C-SPAN So You Can Laugh More

Psychologists at the University of Akron in Ohio asked thirty-three men and women to compare their sense of humour with that of a sibling who had died, and most said they laughed more than their sibs ever had. Well, they certainly laughed more after the sib died, didn't they?

Another great study found that college student volunteers shown what they considered to be a funny movie (I think it was *Nightmare on Elm Street*) had immediate positive changes in their blood vessel function, while those shown a stressful movie (*Your Parents Are Cutting Off Your Money: Tomorrow*) had immediate tightening in their arteries.

Laughter can also help you lose weight. One study estimated that laughing for ten to fifteen minutes a day could burn an extra fifty calories. So go ahead and buy *Why Black People Are Some of My Best Friends* by Barbara Bush, *The Art of Surrender* by Jacques Chirac, and *The Secret of Aging Beautifully* by Bob Dylan. It's an investment in good health.

Copy Your Kids and Lower Your Ambitions

A wonderful study from the U.S. found that the younger a man was when elected governor in his home state, the more likely he was to die early. This finding also holds true for Canadian prime ministers and Nobel Prize winners; that is, the earlier these people achieved their success in life, the more likely they were to die prematurely. So achieve nothing early in life and you will live a lot longer for it. Achieve nothing and you will also kill your parents prematurely so you will get your inheritance a lot sooner, too.

Move to Malta

A guy who's studied happiness for over twenty years has concluded that the "happiest countries" in the world are Denmark (clearly because of the comfortable furniture and the great pastry), Switzerland (chocolate, cheese, and mostly, of course, numbered bank accounts), and Malta (what the hell do they do in Malta besides make crosses?). Next on the list are two countries with tons in common: Ireland and Iceland (I've been to both and I have to tell you, the reason Irishmen and Icelanders seem so happy is probably because they're drunk much of the time.), followed by Ghana (Ghana? You really have to question this guy's methodology, I think.), and finally Canada, but clearly not including Quebec, where the only happy moments they ever have are when the family gets together every Friday night to bitch about the constitution over dinner. He also says, by the way, that to maximize happiness, you should avoid having children. No comment.

If You Don't Have Something Nice to Say, Don't Say It

According to research presented in the *Journal of Personality and Social Psychology,* if you say something negative about someone, there is a strong tendency on the part of the listener to ascribe those traits to you. So if, for some unfathomable reason, you don't like this book, sit on it, OK? It's only going to boomerang on you if you tell someone. I tell you this for your own benefit.

Fool Yourself

If looking older makes you unhappy, as it does many people, a great way to deal with that is to pretend it ain't happening, Jack. A poll for Ortho Pharmaceuticals, for example, published in *USA Today,* revealed that three in four baby boomers think they look younger than their age, and nearly 80 per cent of middle-agers think their faces look younger than those of their peers. Sure, you do, heh, heh, sure you do.

You can fool yourself in other ways, too. Just push the goalposts farther out. That's what most of us do, it seems, because according to that same poll, the older you are, the later you say that middle age starts. People who are thirty to thirty-four say that middle age starts at forty, while those who are already forty-five to fifty think that middle age really only starts at forty-four. They're all wrong, by the way. Middle age actually starts at sixty-four. And a half.

Another good way to fool yourself and benefit from it is to tell yourself that no matter what your mother says, that girl you married is still a catch. A study in the *Journal of Personality and Social Psychology* concludes that people in the happiest relationships tend to see their partners through rose-coloured glasses. You're stuck in anyway, so why not tell yourself it's for the best, eh? Anyway, that's what I keep telling my wife every time she wonders about me. "It's not me, dear. You're just wearing the wrong glasses today."

Do One Good Thing a Day

A study from the State University of New York at Stony Brook published in the journal *Health Psychology* shows that a small boost to the immune system that comes from doing something pleasant can last for up to two days. So go ahead. Start doing a few nice things every day. Put the toilet seat down once in a while, give the squeegee kid a dime once a month for his caring work, don't kick the awful busker's can over for once, and so on. Believe me, you will feel so much better for being so nice. And the new friends you will make!

Lose Your Job

A study from the University of North Carolina suggests that contrary to what you might expect, losing one's job may contribute to a longer, healthier life for some people. Why? Well, I'm sure this is not going to surprise anyone who has ever spent any time in the company of young, happy, unemployed snowboarders, but this researcher concludes that most people are happier when they're not working. Imagine that, eh? Not only that, work can be hazardous, work is often stressful, and work takes time, time that could be spent on exercise and making yourself healthy, which is exactly what I'm sure all those unemployed kids rush off to do as soon as they lose their jobs. So the more you work, the less healthy you may be. I had no trouble convincing my son about that one, of course.

Become a Shrinking Violet

British researchers claim that being submissive and having low self-confidence can reduce the risk of a heart attack, especially in women. I quite agree, and that is why, as a husband very much interested in my wife's health, I pinned this finding to my fridge door. No luck, I'm afraid. My wife ripped it up and, well, I won't tell you the exact words she used, but suffice it to say that a shrinking violet with poor self-esteem would never have used that kind of language. Or tone. Or fists. I wouldn't put much trust in this one, I think.

And the Most Important Advice of All: Don't Feel So Guilty

A British study concluded that people the world over are plagued with guilt about smoking, eating, alcohol use, and exercise, and that that guilt is producing lots of stress. So, folks, accept this absolution from this expert on guilt: Don't feel guilty. It's not worth it. And besides, you're doing your best. Now enjoy your life. And buy my other books.

INDEX

• • •

C

D

E

F

G

H